D1548340

The Guys' Guide to
HASHIMOTO'S

ROCK ROBBINS
of Married to Hashimoto's

www.marriedtohashimotos.com
contact@marriedtohashimotos.com

Praise for
The Guys' Guide to Hashimoto's

"Thank you Rock for writing this much – needed book. You will help save marriages around the world."

Dana Trentini a.k.a. Hypothyroid Mom
Thyroid Advocate and Author

"The Guy's Guide to Hashimoto's is a must read for any man in relationship with a woman diagnosed with Hashimoto's. Rock does an outstanding job of simplifying this complex autoimmune disease by explaining – in easy to understand terms – its impact on a woman, man, and their relationship and what to do about it. Rock is masterful at pulling the veil off one of the most hidden aspects of this much misunderstood disease – that the courageous women who are fighting mightily against this dreadful disorder frequently appear to be perfectly well. I am left smarter, wiser, and more compassionate for having read this book. Thank you, Rock, for this much needed work."

Stephen Conenna, PE
Guy, and author of Use Your Mind to Heal Your Body

"I really do appreciate the work you are doing, my wife has suffered for many years with Hashimoto's and it really has destroyed our lives and marriage. I am desperately trying to support my wife but I'm really struggling myself. It has taken me a long time to realize I have been part of the problem, i.e. I have been causing my wife stress by trying to fix things all of the time, instead of just supporting and loving her, giving her time and space, and just believing in her own instincts - that's why your writing really hit a nerve! Thank you for everything you are doing to help others."

Craig Thorpe
Guy

"I bought this book with the full intention of reading the whole thing myself first before passing it on to my partner to read. I must admit I was a little apprehensive about what would be in it and the advice given.

By one third of the way through I felt very safe in giving it to my partner to read. Rock writes from a place of loving support, decades of experience and a genuine desire to help others support their partner through Hashimoto's.

This is the only book on the market that explains how a couple can best deal with the major health and emotional challenges that can arise from this dis-ease.

My partner found this book to be very informative and full of great links and information that is set out in an easy to understand way.

This is a positive and refreshing look at Hashimoto's from a partner's perspective and provides helpful information to fast track your partner to be the most helpful they can be.

Well done Rock for writing about your insight and experience in a loving and supporting way."

Danielle Pearsall
Thyroid Advocate (Australia)

"Thank you for your many words of wisdom and hope. I am one of those husbands you talk about. I stay in the fight because I know my wife is in there fighting to get out. She is my whole world and I will not let her be beaten by this. Thanks to you we finally have hope."

Brandon Duncan
Guy

The Guys' Guide to Hashimoto's

First printing, November 2016

Library of Congress Control Number: 2016918047
ISBN 978-1-935798-12-5

Rock Robbins
427 East 17th Street, Box 123
Costa Mesa, CA 92627
www.marriedtohashimotos.com
contact@marriedtohashimotos.com

Cover Layout and Design
David Trotter (www.8trackstudios.com)

Interior Layout and Design
Rock Robbins

Photo of Rock
Nigel Skeet (www.nigelskeet.com)

Photo of Stacey
Carissa Boles (www.carissaboles.com)

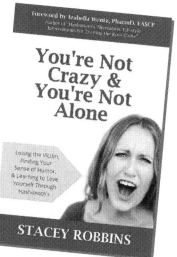

Rock's Disclaimer

This book is my journey as a husband of my Hashimoto's wife. My book is for inspiring and educating men on how to be their best and most informed partner to their Hashimoto's / hypothyroid women. All content is informational only and should not be considered a substitute for consulting your physician regarding medical advice pertaining to your, or anyone else's, health.

I am not responsible for any loss, injury, or damage that allegedly arises from any information in this book. You are responsible for your own health and relationship journey and any actions you take regarding your medical care and your relationships.

All external references represent the views and opinions of those individuals or organizations.

FYI - in this book I often make reference to "your woman", "your girlfriend", or "your partner". These are not to be construed as ownership, as in some kind of non-politically correct cartoon caveman version where you drag "your woman" around by her hair.

I use "your woman" so I don't have to write "your wife/girlfriend/partner" every time – which is just aggravating and tedious to read over and over and over and over.

She is "your woman" the same way you are "her man" in "your relationship."

The Guys' Guide to
HASHIMOTO'S
ROCK ROBBINS

Where the heck is everything?

Introduction

Welcome guys – this is **Rock Robbins,** your host to the adventure of what it's like to have a woman with Hashimoto's in your life.

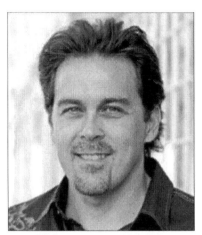

So, if you're a guy and you're reading this – congratulations. That you're even looking at this puts you into the rare category of guys who are trying to understand what your woman is going through.

So, way to go.

May I say that I did not fall into this category until years later in my relationship with my girl, **Stacey**. And let's face it; the "average guy" is probably fine if his girl is going through some health issue, as long as...

1. **He doesn't have to do too much and...**
2. **He doesn't have to think about too much**

If you're like me, I leave a lot of the health issues to my wife as she's just more naturally nurturing than I am. As guys, we have many other things in our life vying for our attention – family, work, friends, finances, sports, cars, (insert yours here). If you're already active in the "help and support your woman" department – awesome for you, keep it up.

9

I got married to Stacey about 27 years ago. Seven years in she got sick and a few years later she was diagnosed with Hashimoto's. It changed our life, because it changed her life. Suddenly I was **Married to Hashimoto's.** (That's my blog, btw, **www.marriedtohashimotos.com**. Check it out)

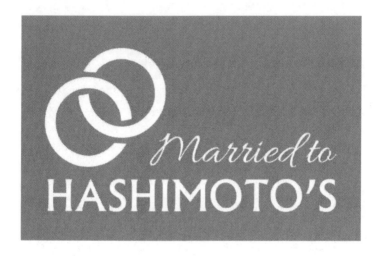

Writing this book has been a pretty amazing adventure for me, literally, as I've been writing this from Florence, Italy on over to San Terenzo, Italy. Italy – a place that was a dream for my wife to bring me and our boys to.

Honestly, with how sick she was in years past with Hashimoto's, a trip like this would not have been possible. Thankfully, she's doing much better, so here we are!

We are by a wonderful ocean area, but I have not gone into the water much. I'm sitting on a built-in bench in the bottom level of a home looking at an internal wall, with a painting on it. It's just the way this crazy house is laid out; I can't even turn around and face the window. I get to take a look at this painting until I'm done with the book...

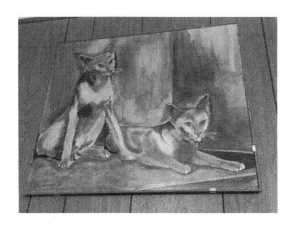

This painting is my inspiration to finish this book, so I can go be with my family and play in the ocean with them! Well, and help make a difference in relationships and families all over the world.

Until then – cats. This is my sacrifice for you.

Ciao,

Rock

Rock Robbins
(San Terenzo, Italy 6/2016)

How to Use the Guys' Guide to Hashimoto's

I'm a lot of things: I'm a deep researcher into whatever subject I'm studying. I'm also an exhausted father, husband, and co-provider who wants the cliff notes on life because, probably like you, I have a lot of other things going on.

So, even though the OCD part of me wants to give you every nook and cranny of my 20 years of experience and many hours of studying, I get it that you probably want the "info I can use now" version. That's what I've put together here. **The Guys' Guide to Hashimoto's** is broken down this way:

Subject – What we're talking about regarding Hashimoto's. Whether it's her moods, energy, stomach, libido... I've got some of the basics subjects covered here to get you started.

Science – The science behind the topic. If you're anything like me, you want to know how the dots are connected between her symptoms and the science.

Suggestions – These are the suggestions that I put together to help you, based on my own Hashimoto's life experience, and accumulated wisdom.

This is not an exhaustive guide on all things Hashimoto's – that's the good news. You're likely already overwhelmed and just want to know what's going on and what you can do about it. I get it.

Yet, this is a little deeper than just a pamphlet too. But we'll talk about this more in the next chapters. If you want to zoom right over to a hot topic for you, go for it. The other chapters will be there for you when you need them.

In the meantime, this guide is here to encourage you and equip you with information you'll need to help this woman you care about who's struggling with a very legit autoimmune disease.

If you have any suggestions or comments about the book, email me at **contact@marriedtohashimotos.com**.

Ready? Let's go...

6 Tips That Will Save Your Time, Your Sanity, and Your Sex Life

Hashimoto's, for you guys who are still learning the ropes, is an autoimmune condition where the body attacks the thyroid. The thyroid controls pretty much everything from weight to moods, from sleep to sex – and about a million things in between.

Even if you only do some of the suggestions I'm about to lay out, it's likely your life will get much better between you and your woman as she grapples with a Hashimoto's diagnosis.

Alrighty then, let's get right to the list...

Tip #1 – Realize that even though she looks "normal", she's not

Here's the thing with Hashimoto's, when it first gets going in someone's body they can seem totally fine on the outside. Things seem okay, but then they start dealing with things like...[1]

- **Fatigue**
- **Brain fog, or fuzzy thinking**
- **Pale / puffy face**
- **Anxiety**
- **Depression**
- **Constipation**

- **Feeling cold**
- **Joint pain**
- **Thinning hair**
- **Low libido**
- **Slowed heart rate**

And those are just some of the symptoms she may have before we enter the exciting world of **weight gain**.

The problem is, in the beginning, we as men may dismiss these things, or hope that they go away like they do with most healthy people. But with Hashimoto's, when untreated, things can steadily move into more and more very un-fun symptoms that just don't "go away".

Tip #2 – Stop acting like this is all in her head

I wish I didn't have to put this here, but even I have fallen prey to the "I feel fine, so you should too" kind of thinking. We get so busy, that when our partner is sick, it cramps our style, and all that we want to get done. If she's looking "normal", it's tempting to say, "Hey! Snap out of it, and let's get back to the fun, and all the things we used to do." Again, with most healthy people, some rest and time is enough to have their bodies repair anything that's going on, but this is no ordinary health issue.

Hashimoto's is basically your body fighting against itself, and attacking the "master" gland in your body, the thyroid.[2] The thyroid's main job is to control metabolism, which is our body's ability to break down food and convert it to energy. The hormones the thyroid creates are essential to proper development of all cells in the human body.[3]

Whoa, let's pause and read that last sentence again, especially the ALL CELLS part. These hormones also regulate protein, fat, carbohydrate and vitamin metabolism.[3]

The reason you're able to sit there and calmly read this book is because your thyroid is working in concert with the rest of your body. Trust me, this is not something anyone wants, and if they do have it, they don't want someone giving them nine miles of bad road on how they're dealing with it.

The whole function of the thyroid can be hard to wrap your head around, so take a look now on **YouTube** for a short **TED-Ed video** about it by **Emma Bryce** titled **"How Does the Thyroid Manage Your Metabolism?"**

I'm a bit of a geek, so I like to think of this like troubleshooting a computer. If the motherboard has something wrong with it, it's not going to matter if all the other parts are sound. Things likely won't work properly for long, if they even work at all. And with Hashimoto's, it can easily be misdiagnosed as other health issues; you can end up doing a LOT of troubleshooting and tests on specific symptoms for a long time before you finally get to the big picture of a Hashimoto's diagnosis.

Quick FYI – thyroid disease alone affects 20% of Americans – that's 1 in 5![4] Of that number, Hashimoto's is the most common cause of low thyroid and affects women ten times more than men.[5]

Trust me, if she could just flip the switch to get back to "normal" she would. She doesn't want to be a drag, not feel well, be stuck wondering what to do, and be frustrated with why her doctor doesn't seem to deal with this effectively (I'll have more on that later).

So, do yourself a favor, **instead of putting that energy of frustration against her, put it toward helping her feel understood, comfortable, and cared for while you both sort out these next important steps.**

Again, this will give you major bonus points for being part of the solution, and not just another reminder that she's broken or crazy.

(When you get a chance, Google search and read **The Power of "I Believe"** [6] by my wife **Stacey Robbins** – it's at her website **www.staceyrobbins.com**. And have your woman read it too. It's a powerful article that will give some important perspective.)

Tip #3 – Don't be a jerk

This goes hand in hand with #2. Sorry to be blunt guys, but we can sometimes be dismissive when someone else is having a health issue, especially with Hashimoto's where a person can seem "normal" on the outside.

"You look fine"

"Why are you just lying around?"

"Maybe if you get up and start moving, you'll feel better."

We can be so sure we're right, and that we know what's going on, **we'll treat people the way we <u>think</u> they are, rather than the way they <u>actually</u> are.**

And it doesn't help us that a great share of our well-meaning primary care physicians push only ONE protocol by saying that this issue is easy to solve just by taking a pill – most of the time it's not.

(See the **Conventional vs. Alternative – What's the Deal?** section for more on this.)

Hashimoto's usually presents itself as one complicated ass-kicking disease. Trust me, if you were going through this, feeling awful with no energy, fuzzy thinking, and pain, you'd have a lot more compassion.

If it helps, imaging the feeling after being kicked in the nuts, and the sickening and aching aftermath of that; then imagine that lingering feeling going for days on end, or months, or years.

You wouldn't want someone getting up in your face and saying…

>**"What's the matter with you?"**

>**"You look fine."**

>**"Just get up and act normal again."**

Tip #4 – Be a part of the team,
it benefits everyone (especially you)

Hopefully you're already onboard with this. But if you've ever seen a family where the mom has been taken out with a bad cold or flu, you know what a big impact that has on the home.

Meals quickly become Dad making cereal, canned soup, or microwave and takeout meals for days. The house becomes a mess overnight. The sports and social schedule gets jacked up if Dad isn't already clued into the regular routine. Hopefully family or friends come to help. Regardless, the impact is felt keenly in the home when the person running the house is taken out with sickness.

Now if you're already getting in there and having her rest and eat good food – awesome. If you're not – pick up the slack in the home, and be an agent of help and peace. It will benefit you in major ways.

The last time I had a major flu where I was taken out for 3-4 days, I remember how my wife kicked into gear and helped me (all while juggling the household, her work, her mother who was in from out of town, and our kids igloo school project that involved oversized marshmallows and a hair dryer).

I was so grateful and impressed by her steady care of me, all without complaining. This is what I try to remember anytime she needs a helping hand or she's feeling sick or depressed.

You have no idea how much it will benefit <u>you</u> to invest in your woman's health – either through caring for the immediate needs, or researching what could help. It's like investing in an account that gets 150% interest – it's worth everything you put in there because the amount of gratitude, and other benefits you'll get from a spouse who knows you have her back.

I'm not saying that that you should do all of this to get sex. But hey, if you're not being an A-hole and you're helping her like crazy, things happen.

Tip #5 – Choose to be Mr. Consistent with whatever version of her shows up

Yeah, this one takes some intention and determination because when a woman is going through Hashimoto's, and the attendant emotional and physical ups and down, you may get...

- **Angry partner**
- **Exhausted partner**
- **Frustrated partner**
- **Thankful partner**
- **Sad partner**
- **"It's all <u>your</u> fault" partner**
- **Fearful partner**
- **"I give up" partner**

Let me put it this way... I have an Italian wife, who's super passionate, creative, and very much human. We have had some amazing times, meh times, and hard times together over our almost 30 years of marriage together; there's no one I love more than her.

One of the things that has served us well throughout the years was my **learning how to hug a porcupine** – or love a wife who is frustrated, angry, and hopeless.

I have had times of really bringing my A game to these scenarios, where I choose to love her even though she's not reflecting that love back to me.

Other times, I've gotten frustrated at her, and basically given her a hard time – not so helpful. Usually I think back to the times when she helped me, and I get back on track.

But heck, even if she hadn't taken care of me – I have a commitment to her that is strong that was truly tested during her many years of whacko symptoms.

So, here's the question to you:

What is your level of commitment to this person?

Because, it could get really gnarly in this process before it gets better. Meds, supplements, and diet changes often don't show benefits overnight so, even if you're on the right track, it still takes time for her body to respond to the good things you're doing.

You should really decide who you're going to be now, 'cause it's likely going to get bumpy, possibly for a long while as you both dial in what works for her.

I'm not trying to scare you, but if you're faint of heart, or in the **"till inconvenience do us part"** type of commitment level, it may not go well for both of you. She's going to need to focus her energy on getting rest, tracking symptoms, food

22

changes, mind issues, and listening to her body to find that sweet spot of what works for her.

Truly, I want you to be there for your woman, the same way I want *me* to be there for my wife. To put any excuses aside (if you have any) and put the time and effort that will be required to get her back to health and wholeness.

Again, this is an investment that will benefit both of you.

We can do it. **You** can do it.

Tip #6 – Know that it's possible to get her health and life back

This is really important. Without hope, it would be easy to get discouraged. So many doctors' visits and tests. Medications and food protocols. Reading thyroid books. Making logs of symptoms and thyroid levels. Taking walks together and talking through how we're doing. Getting the kids on the same page. Making sure you get time to recharge your own batteries.

But for me, I can tell you that it's worth all the work we did to get my wife to where she is now in her health. She has more energy and peace. She knows what works for her food-wise, and what relationships don't add to her life.

This whole adventure is more than just food or pills. You may be thinking,

"Oh joy... there's more?"

Yes, there's more, but that's ultimately a good thing. It's highly likely that some of her prior ways of thinking and living are part of the issue. The truth is that her new "normal" may be very different than what it was before. Different foods, different pace, and a different way of being. What worked back then may not work for this new season.

With Hashimoto's, her body is waving a white flag and saying, through symptoms, "There's something going on! I can't do this the same way anymore!" This is the opportunity to take the cue and adjust accordingly.

And hopefully, through the experiences my wife and I went through, we can short cut you to the quickest road back to sanity, health, playfulness, peace, and even the bedroom.

(Can't click on these? Well, this is just a book. Search online for the title, or go to **www.marriedtohashimotos.com/booklinks** for all of the links listed here, plus more.)

Referenced articles:

1. **Is My Thyroid to Blame? 38 Most Common Symptoms – Dr. Frank Lanzisera**
   http://www.totalhealthmagazine.com/Thyroid-Health/Is-My-Thyroid-to-Blame-38-Most-Common-Symptoms.html

2. **What You Need to Know About Your Thyroid Health – Dr. Joseph Mercola**
   http://articles.mercola.com/thyroid.aspx

3. **Thyroid Hormone – Science Daily**
   https://www.sciencedaily.com/terms/thyroid_hormone.htm

4. **General Information – American Thyroid Association**
   http://www.thyroid.org/media-main/about-hypothyroidism

5. **Hypothyroidism In-Depth Report – The New York Times**
   http://www.nytimes.com/health/guides/disease/hypothyroidism/print.html

6. **Autoimmune Dis-ease: The Power of "I Believe" – Stacey Robbins**
   http://staceyrobbins.com/autoimmune-dis-ease-power-believe

Video Reference:

(YouTube) TED-Ed video "How Does the Thyroid Manage Your Metabolism?" – Emma Bryce
http://youtu.be/iNrUpBwU3q0

My Story

I'm **Rock Robbins** – a husband, dad, tech geek, singer / saxophonist, and now an author. I've participated in many entrepreneurial efforts over the last three decades: Business owner, professional musician/music director, non-profit co-founder, tech writer and coach to couples and men going through hard times in their marriage. If it has something to do with a computer, music, or supporting people, I've likely done it.

About a year ago, the tech company I was working for was sold, giving me a rare opportunity to reassess where I wanted to spend my time and energy. Many men I talked to, who had gone through the same thing, said it opened the door for them to do something they believed in. This book is part of my effort in giving back.

My goal is to shortcut couples who are going through a Hashimoto's diagnosis so that they don't have to go the long and hard way we went.

This is my story of how I got **Married to Hashimoto's**.

First a little back story...

The Early Years

Fresh out of high school, I found myself at my local community college. I wasn't exactly sure what I wanted to do in life, but I was pretty sure that music and computers would be a part of it. I was this tall, trim, Southern California native who was fun, energetic, and passionate. I loved music and played saxophone and sang in local bands.

One day, in one of my music classes at school, I saw her. **Stacey Anne Confalone** came into the classroom. Young, confident, brash, sexy... and so different from many of the other Southern California girls I was used to.

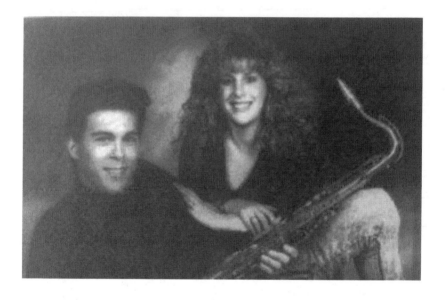

(Our early music promo photo – we had hair to spare)

I liked that this East Coast girl was accessible and open to conversation, unlike many of the aloof girls around campus. She was unlike anyone I had ever met. I mean, she was odd, but in a good way. Heck, I was my own version of weird, so I guess it was a match. I eventually asked her out and that started our adventure together.

Since we were both musicians, we started performing together – first in studio recordings, and later as a musical duo, establishing a professional music career together. We also loved walking and talking, and our relationship grew closer on many levels.

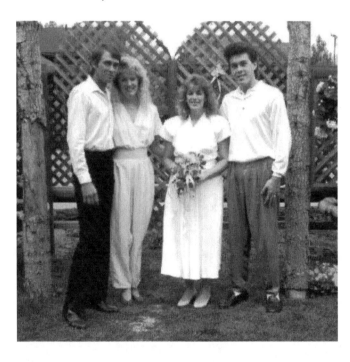

Good god, what a cheesy photo. Check out my classy penny loafers with white socks. Oh well, we were young.

We ended up eloping in 1989 when I was 21, and she was 20. So, that was our wedding photo. We didn't really know the people next to us there very well; we met them in the restaurant lounge where we were playing at the time.

I would like to say that it remained all fun and wonderful, but the first years of our marriage were "bumpy". We were both new to the whole married game and it took time to work out getting used to each other. Plus, I have to admit, I was selfish. It wasn't a pretty process, but right around year seven, our marriage started coming together, and Stacey's health started falling apart.

What The Heck Happened?

There was no shortage of stressful events going on.

- **Our marriage had issues and for a time we were separated**
- **Stacey's parents were in the process of a divorce**
- **She got hit in two separate car accidents**
- **Her grandmother died**
- **Her dad started going through the process of dying**

A whole lot of <u>not</u> fun. It was during this culmination of stress when Stacey's body started having odd symptoms...

- **Skin problems**
- **Dry hair**
- **Joint pain**

- Depression
- Anxiety
- Chronic sinus infections
- Fatigue
- Menstrual issues
- Erratic sleep
- Dizziness
- Brain fog
- Panic attacks
- High sensitivity
- And the one that hits women hard...

Weight Gain!

Really, it seemed that everything just started going down the tubes for her mind and body.

Doctors, Tests, $$$, Frustration, Repeat...

We did what anyone would do in such a situation: we went to our doctor to try to get help. In the beginning, we were trying to deal with all the different symptoms separately. In retrospect, it was a bit like only seeing individual pieces of a larger puzzle, and not being able to see the big picture.

Stacey had begun having stomach issues, so one doctor, thinking it was some kind of bug that needed to be killed, had her take antibiotics.

OK, but after many rounds of antibiotics and six months later, this doctor admitted that he was stumped. We didn't know that you're really not supposed to take antibiotics month after month after month – as it can seriously jack up your stomach.

When one doctor or specialist had tried everything in his or her repertoire, we'd move on to someone else.

After enough traditional doctors couldn't dial her health in, we eventually moved on to alternative doctors and treatments – chiropractic, acupuncture, herbal supplements, meditation, and on and on...

We had so many different prescriptions and bottles of things that had been tried and abandoned. The whole process was really a time, energy, and money-sucking experience. God bless Stacey that she kept on moving ahead – trying different things, asking friends, doing research. As lousy as she felt, she kept moving forward.

Husband of the Year! (Not So Much)

I, on the other hand, wasn't really committed as I could have been. The whole scenario had become just another thing I had to do, so I became more of a passenger on Stacey's crazy health trip. I would sit with her in doctors' offices and they'd review the symptoms... again.

I basically thought that she was already on the case and I couldn't offer anything more. I went back and forth between being supportive and being selfish. I'd drive her to different doctors, but I'd also drive her crazy by being checked out of the reality of her situation. My inconsistency was a big part of the stress on her health and our marriage.

The truth was, she was scared. And she was looking for assurance. Her being sick physically, stirred the pot emotionally. Stacey's Italian family background was full of superstitions, like "If something good comes along, watch out! You're likely going to get hit with something bad." Which played in perfectly with the timing of everything – like I said, our marriage was just getting better, meanwhile the doctors told her she might not live through this, and if she did, she'd likely never have children. This all played perfectly into her "doomed" world view.

In her desperation and pain, she asked me,
"Do you think I'm going to be okay?"

I thought she was just asking for an <u>honest</u> answer.
So, I said, **"Hon... I just don't know."**

I could see from her face, that didn't really help.

She later came back to me and said, **"I know you were just being honest, but can you take some time and come back with an answer that's honest AND encouraging?"**

Yeah, I kind of missed that opportunity.

After thinking it through awhile, I came to her and said,
"I don't know all of what's going on hon – but I'm going to love you back to health."

I gave her great words, but I didn't always follow up with great actions.

Everything Gets Better Now, Right?

After about 15 different doctors and specialists later, we still didn't have an answer. Then one day, while Stacey was out at a music gig, she collapsed in pain. A friend took her to a walk-in clinic where a doctor took labs and then sent Stacey on to the emergency room. We should have had a frequent flyer card for the amount of times we had been to the ER that year.

The doctor called a few days later with the lab results.

"I've got good news, and bad news for you," she said. **"The bad news is that you have Hypothyroidism. The good news is that if you take this prescription, you'll have energy, you'll lose all your weight, and you'll be back to normal within three months."**

Yes! We thought that this was <u>finally</u> it – an actual diagnosis and the road back to health.

That was freaking music to our ears. Stacey jumped in and faithfully took her new thyroid pills, and we waited for life to go back to normal.

Three months later, things hadn't changed for the better. With the new medication, Stacey didn't *lose* weight.

She actually *gained 30 MORE pounds*, until she was at her highest weight of 270. So, unfortunately for us, we found that the standard treatment of thyroid meds didn't take care of the issue.

Because things were getting worse, we had more trips to the doctor. **It took about two more years before we figured out that it was more than hypothyroidism.**

She had an autoimmune condition called **Hashimoto's Thyroiditis**.

It's a disease where the body attacks its own thyroid. Having Hashimoto's can often be MUCH more complicated than the "take this pill and life will go back to normal" assessment we had been expecting.

Here's the before Hashimoto's diagnosis photo, and the after photo, with Stacey at her highest weight.

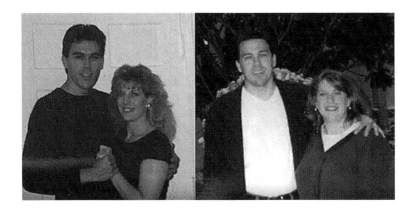

So, our "easy" diagnosis ended up being a complicated disease with multiple issues. Not fun.

While Stacey was dealing with yet another disappointing setback, I really got tested with how committed I was to our marriage – my vows in particular came to mind.

I had to question if I really meant "for better or worse – in sickness and in health" now that I was dealing with the worse/sickness part.

My wife was in a really bad, and complicated health issue that affected EVERYTHING – her weight, her heart, her organs, her appearance... peace, energy, sleep, sex life, fertility, and more.

There was not a lot of information to be had about Hashimoto's 20 years ago. But Stacey didn't give up or take this diagnosis lying down. I wanted to see her well too, so together we went on a mission to understand her condition and find answers. Before long, we were traveling all over the country to different healing centers and health conferences and talking to people all over the world about this Hashimoto's thing.

We found that this condition involved so much more than just physiology.

Many elements played into this diagnosis – it was about stress, food, lifestyle, belief systems, relationships and more.

We have spent the last 20 years, and almost $300,000 diving deep into this dis-ease.

As we unraveled some of the mysteries behind Hashimoto's and took active steps to change our lives, we started getting our life, and her health, *back* – which included having two children – which the doctors said we never would have.

So finally, our life together was moving forward. **But then we learned that pregnancy can greatly affect Hashimoto's**, and after years of progress, we found ourselves in a setback.

Stacey became **depressed, listless,** and even **hopeless-feeling** sometimes.

She found it **hard to concentrate,** and was stricken with **dizziness** so bad that some days, it was all she could do to just get through the day. I was at a loss

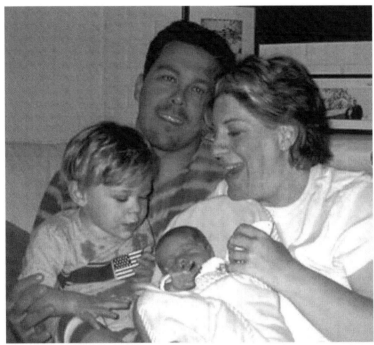

Stacey's pregnancy kicked off another difficult low thyroid season. <u>Bottom line</u>: make sure she has her thyroid levels <u>before</u>, <u>during</u>, and <u>after</u> pregnancy.

Since thyroid levels affect every system in our bodies, you can imagine how important it is for a pregnant woman and her developing child. I would be remiss if I didn't mention a new book that specifically deals with this, it's called...

Your Healthy Pregnancy with Thyroid Disease: A Guide to Fertility, Pregnancy, and Postpartum Wellness
by Dana Trentini & Mary Shomon

(Back to my story)

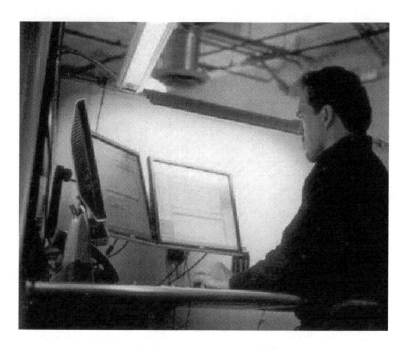

Meanwhile, I was doing my tech job Monday through Friday, and found it to be an escape from the frustrating reality of me not knowing how to help my wife. Sometimes I would come home and all I could do was just eat, relax, play with the kids, and encourage my wife to rest.

Waking Up

The truth is I was waiting for someone else to fix this.

- I was waiting for her to fix it
- I was waiting for the doctors to fix it
- I was waiting for the pills to fix it
- I was waiting for supplements to fix it

And while all of those things matter, it has taken me a long time to realize that...

I can be a part of this healing process.

When I just was in waiting mode, I would go between taking stress away, and then adding to the stress. But as I've been waking up, I realize that **as a husband, I'm a very important part of the equation.**

- **I can help/remind her to take her supplements and mark down her symptoms**
- **I can listen to her, and partner with her on next steps**
- **I can encourage her, when she's down and tempted to give up**
- **I can take the kids out, and let her have time alone or go be with some friends**
- **I can research and be an extra set of eyes on test results, or next step treatment options**

<u>Together</u> we can get to a better place faster. And it's less work to be involved, than it is to resist being involved.

What About You?

- **Are you 100% all in and just need some guidance and information? That's amazing – kudos to you, and I'm glad you're here**

- **Are you half-in, and half-out? Helping sometimes, and causing stress other times? That's honest – so glad you're here**

- **Are you wishing someone else would just fix all this? I understand that too**

I've been in all of these phases. I get it.

This isn't just about Stacey getting her health back; it's been about me waking up. And both of us shifting our expectations from what we *thought* life would be, to accepting what life *is*, and what it can be.

Where You're at Is Not the End

I want you to know that I'm writing this from Florence, Italy – a dream that Stacey and I had when we were first married, but had lost sight of during the dark years of her poor health.

If you are in that hard place too, where you're so busy living in the moment of the pain and frustration that you can't remember the dreams that you have of the future, I want to let you know – there's hope.

Where you're at is only the <u>middle</u> of the story, it's not the end.

Self-Care:
Why It's Important
to Take Care of You

Or, my alternate title, "**Why They Tell You to Put the Oxygen Mask on <u>You</u> First, Before You Try to Help Someone Else During a Flight Emergency.**"

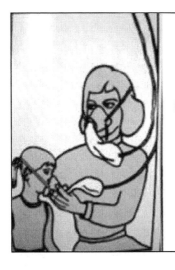

Safety Tip:

Put on your own oxygen mask before helping those around you.

Seriously...
You can't help anyone if you're dead.

The likelihood is that your wife is going to go through different phases of healing:

- **Intensive,** needing more focused attention until she's back on her feet and then...

- **Maintenance**, which requires less intensity. There may be bumps in the road when you have big events like traveling, a job change, kids home for summer, or whatever... that might require some recalibration with her healing routine and household schedule.

But here's the thing - if you're taking care of someone else, you have to take care of yourself. My ultimate advice is to **get some daily rhythms going** that help you to win at being your best.

On a personal note: I've had to learn the hard way that I can't capsize myself with things that don't serve me. It's taken a while to see that I can't drink certain alcohol. I started reacting to it, getting headaches, neck aches and was a wreck the next day.

It wasn't just alcohol. I couldn't drink energy drinks without having the same reaction. So, I'd be feeling like crap because and end not feeling well at work, and then not being able to do what I need to do for my family.

There were other habits too that weren't serving me. Late night video games, TV, or movies meant that I was tired and cranky the next day. Maybe it's getting older, I don't know, but let's just say I'm not 25 anymore and I don't live on an island. Helping my wife heal while her body is out of whack means that I have to make some better decisions for myself.

Here are some suggestions for you to add to your daily routine that can take care of your mind, your body, and your other priorities for the day – and hey, have an open mind. Some of these may not have been in your vocabulary before, but different (let's not call them "desperate") times call for different measures...

When I'm on my A game, some of my rhythms are:

<u>Meditation</u> – My knee jerk reaction to this initially was, "yeah, right… I'm not meditating. I'm not the new age ponytail guy at the local health food store." It seemed un-manly, and just weird UNTIL I found out that one of the most common practices that successful people do regularly is meditate; executives, stock brokers, attorneys, pro athletes, anyone can benefit from it.

<u>Benefits</u>: centering your mind, getting focused, and being more peaceful. Even ten minutes a day makes a difference. If you'd like to know more of the science and why this is good for guys, look up **"A Primer on Meditation"** from the **Art of Manliness website (artofmanliness.com).**

The Honest Guys (thehonestguys.co.uk) have some good general guided meditations.

If that's not your cup of tea, all you have to do is fire up **YouTube** and search for "10 minute meditation" and find something you like.

<u>Yoga</u> – I have to admit, I did not think I would like yoga as much as I do. It's a great way to relax and stretch. It's <u>not</u> require that you wear spandex, just wear some comfortable workout clothes and you'll be fine.

Not sure if yoga is really for men, just look up the **"9 Reasons Why You Should Practice Yoga"** over at **MensFitness.com.**

When I was new to yoga, I tried it in the privacy of my home with my wife (where no one would see me). As I realized the benefits of it and felt more comfortable doing it, I went with my wife to the local yoga where there are many helpful, flexible, and bendy people who will get you into the right class for you.

If you'd rather be awkward in the comfort of your own home, fire up **YouTube** and maybe start with **Man Flow Yoga**. As usual, with the Internet, there are many options to choose from.

Qi-Gong – (pronounced 'Chee-Gong') Again, surprisingly enjoyable and relaxing, this can be an alternative to Yoga. Try looking up **"Morning Qi Ritual with Lee Holden"** on YouTube.

Get Outside and Exercise – It's pretty straightforward. If you need a break, a change of scenery, or just need to get out of where you're working – take a break, go out into the fresh air, stretch your legs, get some sun, and perspective.

A 20-minute walk-run while playing my favorite tunes at lunch, before or after work, and I'm a new man. Really, you can do any exercise you like. Another option, and point of connection with your woman, could be a daily walk together; it's gentle exercise for her, and a time to talk and share about your day.

EFT (Emotional Freedom Technique) – a.k.a. **"tapping"**
I actually use this almost every day before I start my work day. You choose a topic you're trying to work on, and tap at different points on your head and torso. Seemed really odd at first, but it's quite a cool way to refocus your mind, and there's scientific proof that it's effective. [1,2]

It's a bit like hacking your brain. It helps overcome defeating attitudes and beliefs. I personally like **Brad Yates** (he's on YouTube as well), but there a plenty of others out there. **Nick Ortner** has quite a nice program as well.

Top 3 List – I have this big ole master list of all that's in my head. I have a notebook and put that big list in one section. From that, I pick three things that I want to tackle in a day and put that on a separate index card. The reality is that I may only get to one, or I may end up doing those three and more. Having a wife who is healing means there are variables that I can't account for so, flexibility and focus have to go hand-in-hand.

Reading – Seeing something from a different point of view can put some space back into the places in your life that feel tight. Sometimes I pick a book that's of personal interest, sometimes it's something I need to grow in, sometimes it's a book about my wife's condition. Spending 10-20 minutes a day in someone else's wisdom and experience adds to mine.

Some empowering experts who I read/listen to/watch:

- **Robin Sharma** – www.robinsharma.com
- **Brad Yates** – www.bradyates.com
- **Tim Ferris** – www.fourhourworkweek.com
- **Wayne Dyer** – www.drwaynedyer.com
- **Satchin Patel** – www.thelivingproofinstitute.com

Rome wasn't built in a day and you don't have to do all these practices right now. Pick something you like and incorporate it into your life for 5-10 minutes a day for 30 days.

Taking care of you, helps take care of everything and everyone else you care about.

(Can't click on these? Well, this is just a book. Search online for the title, or go to **www.marriedtohashimotos.com/booklinks** for all of the links listed here, plus more.)

Referenced articles:

- **Studies confirm tapping eases emotional, physical and performance issues**
  www.examiner.com/article/studies-confirm-tapping-eases-emotional-physical-and-performance-issues

- **Tapping therapy: curing physical and mental problems**
  www.telegraph.co.uk/lifestyle/wellbeing/7220734/Tapping-therapy-curing-physical-and-mental-problems.html

Referenced websites:

- **A Primer on Meditation – Art of Manliness**
  www.artofmanliness.com/2011/09/07/a-primer-on-meditation

- **General Guided Meditations – The Honest Guys**
  www.thehonestguys.co.uk/general.html

- **9 Reasons Why You Should Practice Yoga – Men's Fitness**
  www.mensfitness.com/training/endurance/9-reasons-why-you-should-practice-yoga

- **Man Flow Yoga YouTube channel**
  www.youtube.com/user/ManFlowYoga

- **Brad Yates (Emotional Freedom Technique / Tapping)**
  www.youtube.com/user/eftwizard
  www.bradyates.com

- **The Tapping Solution – Nick Ortner**
  www.thetappingsolution.com

- **Robin Sharma**
  www.robinsharma.com

- **Tim Ferris**
  www.fourhourworkweek.com

- **Wayne Dyer**
  www.drwaynedyer.com

- **Satchin Patel**
  www.thelivingproofinstitute.com

A Husband's Confession: Lessons from Where I Blew It

I married Stacey in 1989, then seven years later she got a diagnosis, and I was **Married to Hashimoto's**. She didn't get the light easy breezy, take a pill and call it a day version.

She got the **"misdiagnosed for two years, gained 100 pounds, hair failing out, skin bleeding, heart problems, brain toxicity, and we slept in the car outside the Emergency Room night after night for months."**

Yeah, we got *that* version.

This section is sort of my confessional: Where I blew it and what I would do differently if I could go back 20 years.

Seeing as I can't go back in time, one of the best things I can think to do, moving forward, is to live differently and share my honest story of the lessons I learned so that you can have a shortcut. This is not the most flattering portrayal of me, but whatever; if this helps someone get to their health and happiness faster, I'm good with that.

1. Stabilize my family financially

Back 20 years ago, I was not working consistently – that's the first thing I'd address with the younger me.

I'm not sure why that part of me wasn't awake in my 20's like it is for some other guys. Likely, it was that I didn't have a dad growing up and that my mom took care of everything. Whatever the reason, the result was that it made life more stressful for my capable and healthy wife.

I don't know if your wife or girlfriend is like this, but my Stacey is a rainmaker – super, crazy productive. Back then she was a seriously entrepreneurial, headstrong, "make it happen" force of awesomeness.

If a door wasn't open, she could either get someone to open it for her, or she could force it open. (FYI - that's not exactly healthy, but that's a story for another time.) She made it seem so easy when she was feeling healthy and indestructible... so, when I wasn't pulling my weight financially, she didn't wait, she just stepped up and made more money happen by overworking. I was in my own world and was okay with the imbalance while she picked up my slack.

But the reality is that it was too much for her to work my part and her part financially. If we're on the teeter-totter of financial responsibility, and I'm not working my side as a young and capable man, that's a recipe for burnout for her. Which is exactly what happened.

When her Hashimoto's symptoms started kicking in, and she could no longer provide easily, she didn't just go, "Wow, I need some help here Rock. You need to find some work." She *pushed* through those warning symptoms and worked even harder. Unhealthy dynamics on our part, and too much stress, ladies and gentlemen. Way too much stress.

Why do some Hashi's women burn the candle at both ends?

There are some common issues in Hashi's women we've seen over the last 20 years. These ladies are uber-productive, caring, and dynamic. They make life happen and are the heart and soul of their families and communities. One of the hard truths is this: A lot of women we've talked to with Hashimoto's have gone through some kind of abuse, neglect or injury in their childhood.

So, because of that old baggage, they've got their own internal mental circus going on – and one of the main issues they deal with is <u>performing for their worth</u>. That means they'll bypass their inner signals to "stop in the name of health" and keep going so that they can keep being <u>worthy</u> of love.

This is a huge deal for many women. Other unpleasant side-effects include dealing with issues of trust, self-rejection, fear, perfectionism, control, and guilt that sticks like glue. They're almost always "on" – taking care of everybody.

Sound familiar? And my counterpart to that with Stacey was that I didn't have to be "on", because she was taking care of it all. Lots of fun for me: not so much fun for her.

Back to the financial thing...

It's about value. If I value my woman, I'm going to do what I need to do financially so she doesn't have to overdo it and have that extra burden of stress, which affects her mind and body. We both played our parts, but in owning mine, the first bit of advice to the younger me is to get up and start working it. That will provide the context/stability for the next parts.

2. Stabilize my family emotionally

The next bit of advice for my younger self would be – be that steady and unflappable presence when life started going nutty. When all the weird symptoms, doctor visits, confusion, hormone changes and frustration were rocking her world, I didn't need to take it personally and get sensitive about it all. I'd want to be that calm, confident, and protective force in her life. My younger self would have to step up his game and say and do things like...

- "We'll work it out together, hon, you don't have to work it alone"

- "Let's just mark down your symptoms and keep working your health plan"

- "I'll talk to the doctor about why these treatments aren't working, and we'll work the next steps"

- "Alrighty then, which supplements are you avoiding taking today? Let's do that now." (make it fun)

- "You need to rest, I'll take care of the ..."

- "Your (or my) family doesn't seem to understand about Hashimoto's, so I'll fill them in that it's a legit health issue – and that you're not lazy – you just need more time to heal."

You get the idea.

That kind of consistency when the **fit hits the shan** let's her know she doesn't have to be managing everything while she's dealing with brain fog and a life that's turning upside down. And that, my friend, helps with the stress because we're truly being a partner in this, not just going along for the ride.

SIDE NOTE #1: For a while, she may still want to jump in anyway, and try to control things that are over on your side. I'll address that coming up here.

SIDE NOTE #2: This is not permission for you to be criticized by her. Thyroid hormones can make someone be totally out of whack. You can have compassion and not take it personally, but it doesn't mean that you should be treated like crap either.

3. Focus on our priorities

You know how when life is going well, we have the "luxury" to do other things... we can go to the gym, go kayaking with friends, or go golfing, etc...

But when there's some big health event, or an emergency, the circle of our big life pulls in and you focus on your core priorities – make sure you and your family are safe, healthy and whole.

I remember trying to take her out when she was the most sick to do the same things we used to, and she couldn't handle it. The noise of the movies were too overstimulating (anxiety). We'd have to leave the restaurant as soon as she'd start eating (stomach issues). And we'd have to cancel plans or leave early (exhaustion).

So, the next thing I would say to young Rock would be, "Rock, you need to prioritize getting Stacey's health and get her treatment plan dialed in. It may not be easy, but if you take care of this **now,** and invest in her, <u>you'll get back so much of the fun, healthy, and energetic woman you married</u>. Life may not look exactly the same as before, but it's worth your focused investment. If you keep putting her health to the side, it will just lead to a lot of years of frustration with one health issue after another, and bouncing from one doctor to another. It's time to partner with her and take this seriously."

So, I have the perspective now that the shortest distance to her restored health, is to invest the time now, and not wait around and just hope it'll get better by itself.

We are an important part of our wife's healing, and can move it along faster.

4. Change our lifestyle

Again, I'm in front of the younger me. "Rock, next up – some things have got to change...

- First off, you need time for you to recharge and re-center. Make sure you're eating well, do your exercise early morning, or at night after she's asleep, or on the weekend. Get enough rest. It's like those safety drills at the beginning of a flight: make sure you put the oxygen mask on <u>you</u> so that you'll actually be able to help the important people around you.

- No more letting ambitious Stacey clog the calendar with one thing right after another – make margins of 2-3 hours between events. Probably no more of the 1 or 2 nights out a week until she's feeling better. If it looks like there's too much, step in and clear the schedule – even if she protests.

- Make sure she's doing things that are relaxing, fun, and bring her joy. Painting pottery, watching old movies, watching Food Network – whatever. Make sure she gets out with her friends too for perspective.

- Take her out to walk around the neighborhood or at the beach and let her talk, talk, talk and talk some more. Gentle exercise helps her body, and the talking relieves the pressure valve on her head where her thoughts are constantly ricocheting around. She's likely worried a lot about her health and her future and needs some time working it out with you.

- If there are any contentious relationships that are stressing her out, they have to go (or at least be paused) – **even if they're family**! Step in and protect her here.

  "Sorry, Stacey is resting right now and can't talk. What do you need?" Then filter the B.S. out of the conversation and share that, or don't even share that if it's too much.

  The punch line on this, guys, is that you need to take care of you, and you need to help remind her take care of herself.

5. Call in the troops (family and friends)

I'd tell the younger me to work with Stacey to bring our family and friends into the conversation of what's going on health-wise. This is one I wish I had done more proactively with my family. They would dig into her for being lazy because they didn't understand what she was going through. And I'm sad to say I didn't jump in and help them understand like I could have. Not always an easy task, as so many people believe that Hashimoto's is as easy as taking a pill, and boom! You're fixed.

But that's not always the case.

As a recovering Lone Ranger (where I don't reach out and try to do everything myself, or avoid it), I'm finally getting how powerful it is to have a network of people who are there for you and your family's health and wholeness. We both could have used more support that time. So, reach out to your family, your spiritual community, or your network of friends, and bring them into the conversation. There are so many burdens that don't have to be shouldered alone.

6. Get counseling to work on the mental / emotional side

My wife did not start off life as a driven, approval-seeking, Type-A personality out of nowhere – she had a family and life history that shaped her into the person she is. And as her partner, I have my complementary issues that fit with her issues – we're a bit like Yin and Yang, or two puzzle pieces that fit together.

My wife was dealing with Hashimoto's and addressing her physical issues with food, supplements, sleep, and exercise. But that's just one part of the big picture. **It's also important to address the mental issues that run the show behind the scenes. Stacey's not just her symptoms. We had to look at "WHY does she push herself so hard? WHY does she push past when her body is telling her she needs a break?"**

And I had to look at "Why did I let her?"

There's a wonderful doctor and new friend of ours, **Sachin Patel**, a functional medicine practitioner, who shared that a big part of chronic disease can be caused by poor emotional health – usually an emotional or physical trauma that hasn't been released emotionally. That definitely fit what my wife went through growing up.

That's the journey my wife has been on, to work on her whole health – mind, body and spirit. And because life isn't a one-way street when you're married, I had to work on mine, too.

Wait... what? There's more?

Since my wife and I have been dancing together in life in one certain way for such a long while, when one of the partners changes and learns a new dance of health and wholeness, it affects the old dance we've been doing for so long.
So, there's going to be an adjustment time! Woo hoo!!

That's going to mean some stepping on each other's toes as we learn to be in this new dance. My goal is to be gracious, but I have been known to be a pain in the butt in this adjustment process.

So, here's the deal guys: The truth is that so many of us are really great guys married to really great women. We're just in unchartered territory with this Hashimoto's thing. Some of you are already right on task, some of you might be well-intended but asleep at the wheel - like I was, or maybe you're somewhere in between.

It's all good and it's all just a starting point.

The point is that you don't have to live with 20 years of wishing you had done it differently, you can learn from mistakes like mine and take a better road ahead.

As for Stacey and me, we have a great love and commitment to each other – it helped us get past the crankiness, craziness, and hard times that come in every relationship. The commitment was necessary, because there were times when I wondered if we were going to make it. Looking back, I'm so glad we worked through those hard times, because it paved the way for all the good times.

So, there you go. My 20 year retrospective. I hope that this was a helpful perspective from my past that will help your future – now.

What the Heck Is Hashimoto's Anyway?

Before we talk about Hashimoto's, let's do a quick flyby on **what the thyroid does in the body.**

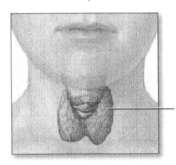

Thyroid gland

The thyroid gland is a butterfly-shaped organ in the neck just below the Adam's apple.

As I mentioned in the introduction, the thyroid's main job is to control metabolism, which is our body's ability to break down food and convert it to energy. The hormones the thyroid creates are essential to proper development of **all cells in the human body.**[1]

If you look at the **American Thyroid Association's FAQ sheet,** it says

"The thyroid gland produces thyroid hormones which help the body use energy, stay warm and keep the brain, heart, muscles, and other organs working normally."[2]

Well, thank God it doesn't control anything important! Sheesh.

There's a reason it's referred to as the **"Master Gland"** or the **"Thermometer of the body"**

The whole process is complicated, but so you're not left in the dark, here is...

The Short Version of the Thyroid Hormone Process
3,4,5

So, the all-important **thyroid gland** doesn't do its job alone. It's a part of the **endocrine system**, which is a bunch of glands that control metabolism, growth, tissues, libido, moods, and sleep.

The **thyroid** works with the **hypothalamus** and **pituitary** glands to control the thyroid hormone levels in the body.

The **hypothalamus** releases **thyroid releasing hormone (TRH)** over to the **pituitary**. With that signal the **pituitary** makes **thyroid stimulating hormone (TSH)** which prods the thyroid make **T4** and **T3** - the main players in this process.

The hormones the thyroid makes are around **90% T4**, and **10% T3**.

What you need to know about **T4** and **T3**:

T4 (a.k.a. Thyroxine) – T4 gets converted by the liver into T3
T3 (a.k.a. Triiodothyronine) – T3, this is where the magic happens. T3 allows the body's cells to create **energy**.

So, it's a complicated system, but that's basically how it's supposed to work in a normal healthy body. When **T4** and **T3** levels are in proper balance, your body's cells hum along nicely.

Ok, now...

What the Heck is Hashimoto's anyway?

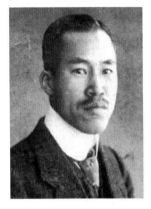

Hashimoto's is named after the Japanese surgeon, **Hakaru Hashimoto,** who discovered it in 1912. [6]

Other names for this disease:

- **Hashimoto's Thyroiditis**
- **Chronic Lymphocytic Thyroiditis**

Hashimoto's is **the most common Thyroid disease in America,**[7] and affects 10% of the U.S. population. It's the first disease that was recognized as an autoimmune disease. [8]

The Basic Definition

Hashimoto's is "a disorder in which the immune system turns against the body's own tissues. In people with Hashimoto's, the immune system attacks the thyroid. This can lead to **hypothyroidism,** a condition in which the thyroid does not make enough hormones for the body's needs." [9]

There are generally three stages of Hashimoto's

From **Hashimoto's Awareness** (a patient education and empowerment non-profit that my wife is on the board of):

"While the allopathic medical community does not generally recognize these stages, we believe they are very helpful in determining prognosis and treatment.

Stage 1: Silent Autoimmunity

In this stage, the body has lost tolerance to its own tissue, but there are no symptoms yet and it doesn't really affect the way that the system functions.

This stage can, however, be identified by lab tests that show elevated antibodies.

People can stay in this stage for years.

This is the best place to begin some sort of treatment because your odds of getting good results are highest. One thing that we know about antibodies is that they are predictive; meaning their presence often warns us about future destruction of that tissue.

Stage 2: Autoimmune Reactivity

In this stage, the destruction of the target tissue has begun. There are elevated antibodies and some symptoms. However, the destruction is not significant enough to actually be labeled autoimmune disease because 70 to 90% of the target tissue has not yet been destroyed.

This stage is where a lot of Hashimoto's patients are.

They may or may not have been placed on thyroid replacement hormone and that may or may not have normalized their thyroid lab results.

However, the destructive autoimmune process is active and is progressing.

This is a very important stage for treating the immune dysfunction because you have a greater chance to slow or stop the destruction of that tissue and slow the progression to other autoimmune diseases.

Stage 3: Autoimmune Disease

This is the stage where Western medicine finally acknowledges that this is an autoimmune disease.

And it takes this long because you need significant destruction of tissue in order to see the destruction with an MRI or ultrasound. Other findings include elevated antibodies, serious and significant symptoms, lab results, and special studies that all confirm a loss of thyroid function.

Unfortunately, this is really late in the game. With Hashimoto's, this is the stage where the thyroid may be significantly damaged.

Most people don't reach this stage before they have been given thyroid replacement hormone because the symptoms have already become so serious that they will have sought out a doctor to help them before they got here." [10]

What causes Hashimoto's?

Doctors ultimately don't know why your body attacks its own thyroid gland. Some scientists think a virus or bacteria might trigger it, and others think it might be a genetic flaw. [11]

Who is at risk for Hashimoto's?

Women, mostly. In the U.S. Hashimoto's affects women 10 times more than men. [12]

What are some other risk factors?

Age – Hashimoto's can happen any time, but usually strikes those who are 30 to 50 years old. [13]

Heredity – Got anyone in your family with other thyroid or auto-immune diseases? That could be a factor.

Other autoimmune diseases - Have **rheumatoid arthritis, type 1 diabetes** or **lupus**? Those also increase your risk of developing Hashimoto's. [14]

Pregnancy – This is big one for women as Hashimoto's sometimes is triggered by pregnancy, so testing for Hashimoto's is important before, during, and after pregnancy. [15]

Viruses/Bacteria – The top three linked to Hashimoto's are **Epstein-Barr Virus (EBV)**, **Yersinia enterocolitica**, and **Helicobacter pylori**. [16,17]

What are the symptoms of Hashimoto's?

To answer this effectively you need to know that there's a difference between **Hashimoto's** and **Hypothyroidism.**

But the real insight that doctors / specialists sometime miss is - **that 95% of hypothyroid patients also have Hashimoto's** [18] **– that's HUGE.**

So, if your woman has **hypothyroidism,** she should check to see if she has **Hashimoto's** as well. It's easy to miss the **Hashimoto's** portion, and that can mean that doctors might only be treating the low thyroid levels (**hypothyroidism**), and not addressing the autoimmune portion, **Hashimoto's** (where your body attacks its thyroid gland).

Missing treating the autoimmune portion can set your woman up for a lot of unnecessary frustration and awful symptoms, possibly for a long time until diagnosed.

I'm going to give you two Hashimoto's symptom lists, the second is more nuanced, and gives a bigger picture. Hang in there.

The **American Thyroid Association** says...

"There are no signs or symptoms that are unique to Hashimoto's thyroiditis.

Because the condition usually progresses very slowly over many years, people with Hashimoto's thyroiditis may not have any symptoms early on" ...

"However, over time, thyroiditis causes slow and chronic cell damage leading to the development of a **goiter (enlarged thyroid)** with gradual thyroid failure, and most patients will eventually develop **symptoms of hypothyroidism**." [19]

Hashimoto's Awareness says...

"Hashimoto's symptoms can vary quite a bit from person to person. People in the early stages may have no symptoms at all.

People in later stages may have lost the ability to function to the point that they can no longer work or care for themselves.

Once it progresses, however, patients begin to experience symptoms that can be felt physically, emotionally, and physiologically.

Hashimoto's typically involves the slow but steady destruction of the thyroid by the immune system.

Eventually this results in a state of **hypothyroidism,** or an under-active thyroid.

However, some patients experience swings from **hypo** or under-active thyroid states to **hyper** or over-active thyroid states before eventually settling into a **hypo** state.

This cycling back and forth can have a big impact on one's ability to function because it causes a whole host of symptoms that are hard to predict and because they are polar opposites.

So, for example, periods of **anxiety, insomnia, diarrhea, weight loss (all hyper symptoms)...**

may be followed by periods of **depression, fatigue, constipation, weight gain (all hypo symptoms)**.

This usually happens because the autoimmune part of the problem has been ignored and focus has only been on the thyroid level.

And the standard practice of increasing thyroid hormone replacement dosages may actually lead to making these types of swings more intense.

As a result, Hashimoto's Awareness advocates early intervention and an approach that involves more than just prescribing thyroid replacement hormone, but also addressing the autoimmune side of the equation.

At its root, autoimmune disease is a disease of inflammation.

And everyone has 'triggers' or things which make this inflammation worse.

Some of the most common are gluten, dairy and soy proteins, stress, blood sugar imbalances and exposure to environmental toxins." [20]

Since Hashimoto's often leads to some being **hypothyroid**, let's look at that definition of that.

> **Hypothyroidism** – "… also known as underactive thyroid, is a condition where the thyroid gland does not create enough of a thyroid hormone called thyroxine." [21]

What are the symptoms of Hypothyroidism? [22]

- **Fatigue, feeling "wiped out"**
- **Sensitivity to cold (cold hands and feet)**
- **Require excessive sleep**
- **Gain weight easily, despite diminished appetite**
- **Goiter (swelling of the thyroid gland. It may be visible on the neck. It can also affect breathing and swallowing)**
- **Neck and back pain**
- **Constipation**
- **Depression**
- **Headaches which are worse in the morning and improve throughout the day**
- **Dry / thinning hair**
- **Dry skin**
- **Heavy menstrual bleeding or irregular periods**
- **Hoarse or raspy voice**
- **Yellow skin**
- **Slower thinking**
- **Slower speech or movement**
- **Slow heart rate**
- **Infertility**
- **Intestinal problems including bloating and heartburn**

- **Osteoporosis**
- **Hypoglycemia**
- **Neuro-degeneration (nerve damage and death of neurons found in Parkinson's, Alzheimer's and Huntington's disease)**

What are the complications of Hashimoto's?

One fourth of Hashi's people may have **chest pain** and/or **joint pain**. Plus, there's an increased risk of **heart disease**. [23]

Myxedema - A rare, life-threatening condition can develop due to long-term hypothyroidism as a result of <u>untreated</u> Hashimoto's disease. Its signs and symptoms include intense cold intolerance and drowsiness followed by profound lethargy and unconsciousness. [24]

How is Hashimoto's treated?

It depends on what's going on.

Here's what the **American Thyroid Association** says... "Patients with elevated TPO antibodies but normal thyroid function tests (TSH and Free thyroxine) do not require treatment." - This means that someone can have Hashimoto's show up on tests but not be hypothyroid (having low thyroid levels) or have any low thyroid symptoms.

For those patients with overt hypothyroidism (elevated

TSH and low thyroid hormone levels) treatment consists of thyroid hormone replacement" [25]

That means that if she has low thyroid level symptoms, she'll be taking a thyroid replacement.

Which specific thyroid replacement is appropriate depends on what she specifically needs. Treatments for this complicated disease really need to be worked out with a competent medical practitioner.

The choice of her doctors and specialists is a hugely important part of your woman's health team – which also includes you on the home front. She's going to need support to work the plan that the team lays out. That's why it's so important to find the right doctor who will not just dispense medicine, but will listen to you and her if things don't seem to be going right as you're executing your plan.

More on that later in the **"Conventional vs. Alternative – What's the Deal?"** section.

Can Hashimoto's be cured?

I want to tread lightly here because this gets into the different camps of thought. But I also don't want to avoid answering this directly. So, here we go...

- There are some that will say **no**, there is no cure for Hashimoto's – only management of thyroid levels.

- There are still others that will say, **yes**.

- And **yet others that won't use the word "cure" but they say you can go into "remission."**

   From what I've seen so far, I personally think remission. That's just my opinion.

And then, **there's the emotional / mind game** – in that if someone believes that there's no hope of getting better, they are likely to get resigned to one treatment option, probably feeling like crap, and saying "oh well, I can't do anything else. This is how it will always be."

Don't let her settle for that.

<u>So, is there hope?</u>

Hell yes, there's hope!

I know many people with Hashimoto's living a healthier and happier life who were sick and frustrated before – that includes my wife.

I definitely believe anyone can get better if they keep pushing to find what works for their situation. No one needs to be resigned to just feeling awful. You may have to work at finding the right doctor and treatment, but it's worth the effort.

Hope is what I want to leave you and your Hashi's woman with.

Because my wife and I were hopeless at times too.

Thankfully, we're in a much better place now.

(Can't click on these? Well, this is just a book. Search online for the title, or go to **www.marriedtohashimotos.com/booklinks** for all of the links listed here, plus more.)

Referenced articles:

1. **Thyroid Hormone**
   https://www.sciencedaily.com/terms/thyroid_hormone.htm

2. **American Thyroid Association's FAQ Sheet**
   http://www.thyroid.org/wp-content/uploads/patients/brochures/ThyroiditisFAQ.pdf

3. **American Thyroid Association's FAQ Sheet**
   http://www.thyroid.org/wp-content/uploads/patients/brochures/ThyroiditisFAQ.pdf

4. **American Thyroid Association's FAQ Sheet**
   http://www.thyroid.org/wp-content/uploads/patients/brochures/ThyroiditisFAQ.pdf

5. **Thyroid Gland**
   http://www.yourhormones.info/glands/thyroid_gland.aspx

6. **How Your Thyroid Works**
   http://www.endocrineweb.com/conditions/thyroid/how-your-thyroid-works

7. **What You Need to Know About Your Thyroid Health**
   http://articles.mercola.com/thyroid.aspx

8. **Hakaru Hashimoto: 1881-1934**
   http://www.healio.com/endocrinology/thyroid/news/print/en
   docrine-today/%7B7429d42f-c45f-4de2-a312-
   e9ba9f6cc860%7D/hakaru-hashimoto-1881-1934

9. **Hashimoto's Thyroiditis Overview**
   http://www.endocrineweb.com/conditions/hashimotos-
   thyroiditis/hashimotos-thyroiditis-overview

10. **Hashimoto's Thyroiditis**
    https://en.wikipedia.org/wiki/Hashimoto%27s_thyroiditis

11. **Hashimoto's Thyroiditis**
    http://www.webmd.com/women/hashimotos-thyroiditis-
    symptoms-causes-treatments

12. **Three Stages of Hashimoto's**
    http://www.hashimotosawareness.org/3-stages-of-
    hashimotos

13. **Hashimoto's Disease Causes**
    http://www.mayoclinic.org/diseases-conditions/hashimotos-
    disease/basics/causes/con-20030293

14. **Chronic Thyroiditis (Hashimoto's Disease)**
    http://www.nytimes.com/health/guides/disease/chronic-
    thyroiditis-hashimotos-disease/risk-factors.html

15. **The National Institute of Diabetes and Digestive and
    Kidney Diseases: Hashimoto's Disease**
    http://www.niddk.nih.gov/health-information/health-
    topics/endocrine/hashimotos-disease/Pages/fact-
    sheet.aspx#sup1

16. **Hashimoto's Disease: Risk factors**
http://www.mayoclinic.org/diseases-conditions/hashimotos-disease/basics/risk-factors/con-20030293

17. **Hashimoto's Disease: The Danger of Thyroid Antibodies and Pregnancy**
http://hypothyroidmom.com/hashimotos-disease-the-danger-of-thyroid-antibodies-and-pregnancy

18. **Hashimoto's Disease: The Infection Connection**
http://hypothyroidmom.com/hashimotos-disease-the-infection-connection

19. **Which Viruses Can Trigger Thyroid Autoimmunity?**
http://www.naturalendocrinesolutions.com/articles/which-viruses-can-trigger-thyroid-autoimmunity

20. **Chronic Thyroiditis (Hashimoto's Disease) In-Depth Report**
http://www.nytimes.com/health/guides/disease/chronic-thyroiditis-hashimotos-disease/print.html

21. **American Thyroid Association**
http://www.thyroid.org/hashimotos-thyroiditis

22. **Symptoms of Hashimoto's Disease**
http://www.hashimotosawareness.org/how-hashimotos-is-diagnosed/symptoms-of-hashimotos-disease

23. **What is hypothyroidism? What causes hypothyroidism?**
http://www.medicalnewstoday.com/articles/163729.php

24. **Is My Thyroid to Blame? 38 Most Common Symptoms**
    http://www.totalhealthmagazine.com/Thyroid-Health/Is-My-Thyroid-to-Blame-38-Most-Common-Symptoms.html

25. **Autoimmune diseases fact sheet**
    http://www.womenshealth.gov/publications/our-publications/fact-sheet/autoimmune-diseases.html

26. **Hashimoto's Disease Complications**
    http://www.mayoclinic.org/diseases-conditions/hashimotos-disease/basics/complications/con-20030293

27. **American Thyroid Association**
    http://www.thyroid.org/hashimotos-thyroiditis

Related articles:

- **Hypothyroidism vs. Hashimoto's:
  what's different and what's similar?**
  http://www.stopthethyroidmadness.com/hypo-vs-hashis

Conventional vs. Alternative – What's the Deal?

So, there was a time, a long, long time ago, when doctors used to come to your home.

WHAT!? Are you kidding me?

I'm telling you, it's true. It was called a "house call."

Doctor Abernathy would come to the house and check in on sick little Timmy.

He'd put down his cool 1950's black doctor bag at the foot of the bed and start talking.

"So, how you feeling today, champ?" he'd ask, looking down smiling.

"Not so good." Came the weak reply. The doctor turns briefly to glance at the boy's mother's worried eyes. He winks.

"Sit up, please."

The doctor pulls a thermometer from his breast pocket and slips it in Tim's mouth. He then puts his stethoscope on and listens, pausing at different points on Timmy's chest and back.

"Did you hear about the Andersons?" The doctor says casually, taking the thermometer out. "You know they have a new puppy."

"What? Really?" Timmy's eyes widen and he's decidedly more energetic than he was a few seconds ago.

"Yep," the doctor leans closer. "Too bad you're not feeling well."

Timmy slouches a little bit, staring out the window, then announces...

"I might not be so bad. Actually, I'm feeling a lot better."

Mom raises an eyebrow, a faint smile on her face.

A few more pleasantries and the doctor is off to visit his next patient.

Quaint scene, isn't it?

A doctor who takes the time to check on you and consider all of what's going on in your life.

Times have changed.

But even though they have, you can still find a health practitioner who has these three qualities: **knowledge, time, and care.**

Here are the two routes that you're going to find yourself considering:

Conventional – also known as Western, mainstream, allopathic and standard. This is the **"go to the doctor, get a test, get a prescription, and take a pill"** routine.

And then there's...

Alternative – also known as Eastern (but not exclusively), holistic, and natural/naturopathic. This is the **"go to a naturopath / doctor / acupuncturist / chiropractor / nutritionist / energy worker / healer, get a protocol that may include vitamins / minerals / supplements / food plan / lifestyle changes"** routine. In my experience, it usually involves drinking something that tastes disgusting, because it's supposedly really, really good for you.

The Power of You

Now, before we dig into doctors, practitioners, and meds, I want to share with you something so VERY important for you and your woman on her health journey.

I dare say...

<u>**This is the most important part of the book.**</u>

Ok, hopefully I have your attention. Here's an "A-ha!" moment that will likely save both of you years of frustration, sickness, and money.

Ready?

First off - this is *her* healing journey, and it's ultimately up to her to find out what works for her. However...

You, my friend, are probably the most important person on her health team.

It's true. Here's why...

When I look back on what my wife and I went through, I realize now that if I had truly partnered with her in this effort, we could have probably shaved off maybe 10+ years or more of just "ok" health for her, and she could have realized her health faster, and had a more vibrant life.

THAT'S how important *you* are in this journey.

I was not plugged into this process for many years, so my wife had to do work of researching, making a plan, engaging health practitioners, taking supplements, doing exercise, and taking time to rest and heal – mostly by herself.

The Power of Two

If you've ever done a workout program on your own, you know how easy it can be to just blow it off if you feel tired, uninspired, or down. But if you have a workout partner, who's going to meet you every day and help you keep your sights on the goal, there's a much higher chance you're going to push past your excuses and get your butt off the couch and do the workout.

That is the **power of partnership**. Marriage, or a committed relationship, is a very powerful thing when harnessed. We get the benefit of our combined strengths.

My wife knows me, my fears, my hopes, and my weaknesses. When she sees me floundering, she can step in and remind me of who I am, and what I'm trying to do in the world.

So, when it comes to her health, and how important it is to her, to us, and to our family, I can step in and help her keep moving; I can help her keep taking those supplements, help her review her meds and how her tests look, and help her keep life more simple and peaceful so that her health is moved forward – which helps our whole family.

Of course, you can't <u>make</u> her do anything – this is her journey. But when your harness your power together toward her getting well, and make that your intention together – good things will happen quickly.

Keeping the Goal in Mind

So, who/what are the best practitioners / meds / supplements / programs?

The answer to that is – <u>whoever and whatever works best for her</u>.

Sorry, that's kind of an aggravating answer, but it's just the reality.

Remember, there's really no one size fits all solution with Hashimoto's. Every person's body is different, and the treatment plan can be very different from woman to woman.

The goal here is to keep in communication with each other, and your doctor as you try a medicine, diet, supplement, exercise, or protocol. This is where the persistence and patience will come in to assess if something's working or not.

If it works well, great – take note of that. Then, keep moving and work on another aspect. If you're just starting out, the goal of just having her feel good or near normal will be the focus.

You're going to have regular life going during all of this, so it will be easier for you both if you make a day where you can both sit down and assess how she's doing, plan your week, and what you're going to work on.

Whose Responsibility Is It to Find out What Works for Her?

It's both of yours.

You can work with your doctor or practitioner, and they can make recommendations, but you guys are responsible to work it, assess it, and report back.

A **health log** is a great idea for tracking...

- How she feels overall
- Current medications and supplements
- Blood test results
- Exercise plan
- Energy level
- Stress level
- Weight
- Mood

Anything you want to track, write it down, or enter it in your computer. Then, you can look back, see patterns and get the big picture – this will help you at your doctor appointments too.

Take time to make regular notes daily or weekly. Because if she's not feeling well, or her brain is unclear, she might not remember later.

I know that I wouldn't remember those details, and I don't have Hashimoto's messing with my brain, so write those down so you can refer to them later.

(As I write this a new app is coming out that helps with this, it's called the **Autoimmune Citizen Science App**. It will not only track symptoms and levels, but there's a community element, and looks like there will be practitioner lists and really, a lot more. They're funding it now, but it's already being backed by some big names in Hashimoto's. This looks really cool, and I will be jumping in and putting money towards it. If you're like me, I find that guys often like having some technology involved to give them something to DO towards the goal. This will be a great help if we work it and help her track symptoms, foods, moods, etc. Check out more at **joinaics.com**)

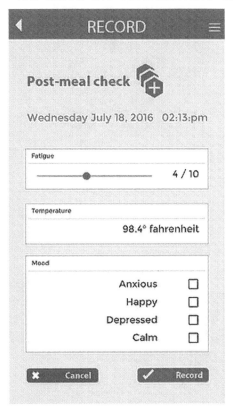

What If Something Isn't Working?

If you've really tried it, and she knows it's not helping, move on to the next thing. Don't waste your time arguing with your practitioner (conventional or alternative) when you know you need to move on.

What will help her is still out there. Keep searching.

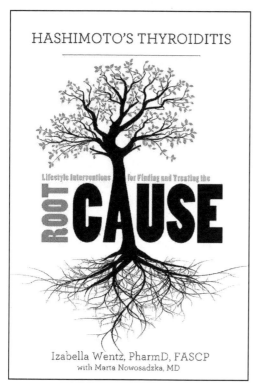

HASHIMOTO'S THYROIDITIS

Lifestyle Interventions for Finding and Treating the

ROOT CAUSE

Izabella Wentz, PharmD, FASCP
with Marta Nowosadzka, MD

Trust me, when you find something that clicks, and she has more energy, or just feels more normal – you will be glad you were consistent and persistent.

This is a good time to introduce **Dr. Izabella Wentz, Pharm D.** – Author of "**Hashimoto's Thyroiditis: Lifestyle Interventions for Finding and Treating the Root Cause.**"

She and her husband, **Michael,** are dear friends and are making a huge difference in the world by helping people find the ROOT cause of their Hashimoto's, so that they not only feel better, but they can even put Hashimoto's into remission (as in you no longer have symptoms and feel like a normal person again).

We were also honored that she wrote the foreword to Stacey's book, **"You're Not Crazy and You're Not Alone"**

Izabella's story as a medical student who got Hashimoto's and found conventional treatments weren't giving her relief from her symptoms – severe stomach issues, fatigue, forgetfulness, joint pain, and hair loss. She ultimately researched and created a treatment plan that helped her find her root cause of Hashimoto's. Her book shows others how they can find their own root cause and get back to health. It's an amazingly informative, inspiring, and hope giving book.

We highly recommend it. Oh, and it's also a **New York Times best seller** too. Congrats Izzy!

Now, back to our regularly scheduled program...

My Story

When we first started this whole Hashimoto's thing, we did the first option – **"go to the doctor, get a test, get a prescription, take a pill."** Stacey was given a pill for high cholesterol, another pill for pain, another pill for anxiety, another pill for infections, another pill for sleep, and another pill for weight loss.

Every individual symptom was being treated individually.

The interesting thing is this, all of those symptoms she was being treated for individually, are actually a composite of a thyroid issue. Many miss the Hashimoto's diagnosis because it can look like a lot of other common issues. With the help of a doctor, we eventually weaned her off of those other meds and put her on thyroid medicine.

If one thyroid pill could replace all the other medicines she was taking before, it would have been great. The standard treatment Stacey was on may have worked for others, but it didn't work for her.

Stacey, who was raised in a family where there were conventional doctors, and alternative practitioners, was exposed to both modalities.

Plus, her crazy Italian family was one of those...

> *"You have a headache?*
>
> *Stick out your tongue.*
>
> *Hmmm...*
>
> *You have to poop"*

...kind of families.

So, when the conventional wasn't the whole answer to her thyroid issue, we went down the alternative route.

We went to **nutritionists, acupuncturists, naturopaths, chiropractors, kinesiologists, reiki masters, Jin Shin Jyutsu practitioners, healers, energy workers,** you name it – we did it. And it was expensive.

Now for me, I was raised in a conventional approach, so a lot of this alternative stuff seemed like crazyville and an unnecessary expense. It took a lot of time, it sometimes took a lot of money, and it didn't always work.

But, sometimes it did.

I couldn't deny that there was effectiveness in both areas. Both took having your brain engaged. And both took some trust.

That picture I painted in the beginning of the doctor with knowledge, time and care, doesn't always just fall into just one camp, or with just one person.

We developed a team of people, with different strengths, to help Stacey to deal with her health. That's why I want to encourage you guys to get the help your woman needs and realize that it could fall in one or both of those camps.

For me, I was really stuck in my judgement about alternative treatments. At the same time, I was really pissed at some of the bumbling and pain that Stacey went through with the conventional side; sometimes, it was like having The Three Stooges as her doctors.

She was told by the medical professionals, **for two years**, that her issues and symptoms were all in her head, all while we're watching her body totally freak out with crazy symptoms.

So, while things were very different in the 1950s with little Timmy, they were also very different in the 1990's – and we had to learn a lot about Hashimoto's through our own experience, research, and trial and error.

We tried the standard treatment that our standard doctor recommended. He prescribed **Synthroid** for 3 months and we were told she'd feel better and lose weight by then.

What happened? Well, she...

- Gained 30 more pounds!
- Had trouble swallowing
- Had itchy skin
- Had problems with swelling

Those symptoms are a sign that something's not right people!

Now, that's just our story. Remember, everyone is different. What worked for my wife, may not be what works for your woman. Again, the goal is to as find out what does work. FYI - there are some people who do well with Synthroid, but the point is, **other supplements/medicines were not even presented as an option –** *not cool.*

I've included some links about other thyroid replacement options. There's quite a menu of supplement options, many more than just the <u>one</u> Synthroid option. **I've found that there are some <u>14</u> other thyroid supplement medications that are options – right now, other than Synthroid.**

It was very cyc opening that these weren't even presented. And since feeling well is SO important to everything else you're both trying to do in life, you want to be clear on ALL your options.

This time we're living in now is an amazing time to be dealing with this diagnosis. Because **we have the best of both worlds –** of the conventional, and the alternative, that have come together to make dealing with Hashimoto's, and maybe even healing Hashimoto's, a possibility that is available to us and the women we love.

Rock's Rant

I gotta tell you, after writing all that, I'm reflecting on all that we've gone through, and I'm kind of pissed. My wife was given the run around, and told that her symptoms were all in her head for a loooong time.

And because I trusted the doctors, more than I trusted my wife, I believed them and was regularly dismissing her remaining symptoms.

There's a particular thing I want to spare you since we learned it the hard way, and I want to remind you of this simple truth:

Knowledge is Power

Some conventional doctors test for thyroid levels, and very often they will only check for **TSH (Thyroid Stimulating Hormone)**. Here's the problem...

<u>It's bigger than just TSH</u> – The standard reference range for TSH doesn't give the whole picture on thyroid function, but many conventional doctors use this as the definitive test of how well her thyroid is working.

> **What's the issue?** The appropriate TSH level is in dispute – some alternative doctors believe the range is too wide and based on out-of-date research. **Yet blood test companies often use this old reference range.**
>
> The problem is that people may be "in range" in their **TSH, and still feel poorly and have frustratingly awful symptoms.**

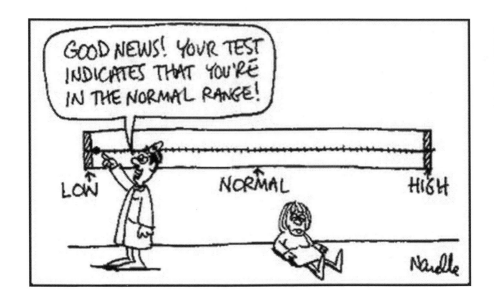

The old wider **TSH** ranges can go from **0.2 - 5.0** (which you may see as "normal" range on an blood test that has these older standards)

After 2003, the **American College of Clinical Endocrinologists (AACE)** had a new recommended range. Here's the relevant quote from their 2003 newsletter...

> "Until November 2002, doctors had relied on a normal TSH level ranging from .5 to 5.0 to diagnose and treat patients with a thyroid disorder who test outside the boundaries of that range.
>
> Now AACE encourages doctors to consider treatment for patients who test outside the boundaries of a narrower margin based on **a target TSH level of .3 to 3.04. AACE believes the new range will result in proper diagnosis for millions**

**of Americans who suffer from a mild
thyroid disorder, but have gone
untreated until now."**

Not sure what happened behind the scenes, but the range later went back out to the wider range. Endocrinologist politics? Maybe.

But the impact of that older wide range can result in conventional doctors declaring symptoms a "mental issue," and prescribe anti-depressants and anti-anxiety medicine. Being told you're fine, when you're suffering, often leaves patients feeling sick and crazy. This is what happened with my wife.

Which brings me to another point...

Some doctors don't like when you challenge their treatment plan with pesky symptoms like...

- She feels tired
- She feels awful
- Her hair is falling out
- Her skin is acting strange
- Her sex life is almost non-existent

If that's your reality, you need to maybe consider getting another doctor, endocrinologist, or consider a more "alternative" specialist who is aware of these tighter ranges, and has more than one tool, Synthroid, to use for your woman.

A very common experience is that **she may be treated as only her lab value, and not as a whole person.**

I mean, what's the goal?

The goal is to have your women feel better, have energy and re-enter the world of the living. Not have her drag around life like a zombie, going "well, at least my doctor says I'm in range."

My wife's book, **You're Not Crazy & You're Not Alone**, specifically shares how she dealt with doctors who misdiagnosed, and other family members (like me) who weren't supportive.

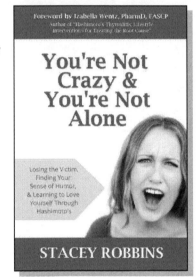

This book is a game-changer for your woman and will help her to be empowered during times like those.

Also, take a look at **Dr. Izabella Wentz's "Top 6 Recommended Blood Tests"** on the web to find out more about what a full thyroid blood panel looks like, and how to get it. Not everything may be covered by your insurance, but it's worth even paying cash for it so that you, and your practitioner, can know the full picture of what's going on.

<u>Pro tip</u>: get and keep copies of ALL her blood tests so you can see, and track her thyroid and TSH levels. As she starts to feel better, you'll be able to see what changed and what works for her.

What if my insurance doesn't cover a different doctor/practitioner, a special thyroid test, or different medicines?

Great question, and very practical. I get it. We may not have the same resources as someone else.

I would work with what I have available first.

Most standard doctors prescribe **Synthroid,** which is often covered by health insurance plans. If that works for her and she feels good on it, you're good. The thing you need to keep in mind is that there are some who don't do well on **Synthroid**.

I was contacted by a woman who had been on a thyroid medicine for five years. She was not feeling well most of that time! Her doctor said she was "in range" and sent her away every year, even though she didn't feel well.

She finally <u>fired</u> her endocrinologist, and was starting another medicine with another doctor who gave her more options. It kills me that she waited that long. But she wanted to trust her doctor's advice, so she put up with feeling sick for <u>years</u>.

And then, if that weren't bad enough, my wife and I got to hear the story of another women, a nurse practitioner, who also was on Synthroid and was resigned to not feeling well - **for 20 years!** And that's a medical professional!

I don't want <u>any</u> woman feeling that bad for that long when there other practitioners who have more experience and "tools" in their toolbox.

There are many women suffering in this type of scenario, and as a result, marriages, couples, and their families are suffering too.

Don't let your woman settle for feeling terrible!

Speak up when it's not going well.

Keep pushing forward to find what works for her.

Quick disclaimer

I believe in modern medicine. It's amazing and it has its place in the world helping people. I've had times where I've dealt with issues, and had my standard doctor work with me and, BOOM, it's resolved.

Also, I believe that most doctors are out there trying to help folks and do what they feel is best for them.

All that being said, I think the reason why there's an "alternative" medical field is because sometimes the standard medical practices fall short, and the alternative is there to fill the gap.

It's an unfortunate reality that some practitioners, treat symptoms or lab values, and don't treat the whole person. That's why it's so important for us to keep moving forward, own our health journey, and report any issues right away so that we can get that important feedback from our medical team.

But it may happen that sometimes you find a doctor or practitioner, standard or alternative, which may not be a fit. Don't worry about it. Release them, and move on. The right person and treatment is out there. Keep moving forward.

IMPORTANT: Any changes to her thyroid medication can take 4-6 weeks to take full effect, so do NOT have her go quickly go on or off meds without her practitioner doing regular blood test and assessing her.

There can be seriously dangerous side effects, so be patient, and carefully work with your doctor when adjusting these, or trying new medications.

I'm still working with my wife to fine tune her meds, supplements, exercise, and rest. New seasons require different adjustments.

Her quality of life is worth the work.

It blesses her, it blesses me, and it blesses our family, and beyond.

Suggestions

- **Own your part of the partnership in her health** – you are an important part of the team!

- **Be open to both the conventional and alternative options** – her answers may lie in one or both places.

- **Do regular research** – Even 10-15 minutes a day will help you and her get more on top of what needs to be done, so you can be a better partner to whatever health practitioners you choose.

- **Meet regularly together and examine how she's doing** – this is where that symptom log is crucial.

Check on how she feels, her energy, her symptoms, her weight, her clarity of thinking.

How's the doctor/practitioner doing? How do her labs look?

- **Keep being that awesome support for her –** when she's tired, confused, brain foggy and weary.

(Can't click on these? Well, this is just a book. Search online for the title, or go to **www.marriedtohashimotos.com/booklinks** for all of the links listed here, plus more.)

Related articles:

The TSH Normal Range: Why is There Still Controversy?
https://www.verywell.com/tsh-normal-range-endocrinology-controversy-3232900

What To Do If Your TSH Is "Normal" And You Are Anything But!
http://thyroidpharmacist.com/articles/what-to-do-if-your-tsh-is-normal-and-you-are-anything-but

Which Is The Best Thyroid Drug For Hypothyroidism?
http://hypothyroidmom.com/which-is-the-best-thyroid-drug-for-hypothyroidism

Hashimoto's: Why Do I Feel Like Crap on Synthroid?
https://www.hashimotoshealing.com/hashimotos-why-do-i-feel-like-crap-on-synthroid

Why Doctors Don't Like Knowledgeable Patients
https://www.verywell.com/thyroid-patients-effect-on-doctors-3231606

Functional Medicine Approach to Healing Hypothyroidism
http://hypothyroidmom.com/functional-medicine-approach-to-healing-hypothyroidism

For the conventional take, check out...

The American Thyroid Association's page on Hashimoto's:
http://www.thyroid.org/hashimotos-thyroiditis

Ingredients in Synthroid
https://www.drugs.com/pro/synthroid.html

What's Going on with Her Stomach?

I thought it was going to be an easy section to write. Oh, how wrong I was.

It's been a mind-numbing exercise to read all the stomach/gut issues that can affect someone with Hashimoto's. I don't know why I'm surprised, it was the main symptom my wife dealt with.

So, here's my attempt to boil it down to the basics. See the referenced articles and additional resources section if you want to dive deeper.

Let's do a flyby on the science.

The Science:
The stomach plays a big, like <u>really big</u>, role in Hashimoto's in that 70-80% of the autoimmune system is in the stomach.[1]

Since Hashimoto's is an autoimmune disease, it's no small deal when there are problems in her gut.

The most common <u>Hashimoto's</u> gut-related symptoms: [2]

- Acid reflux
- Nutrient deficiencies
- Anemia

- Leaky Gut (Intestinal permeability)
- Food sensitivities
- Gum disorders
- Hypoglycemia

Then there are the typical <u>hypothyroid</u> symptoms:

- Weight gain
- Cold intolerance
- Hair loss
- Fatigue
- Constipation

Let's talk about a few important ones:

Food sensitivities – one of the things that cannot be understated is the fact that <u>we are affected by what we eat</u>. Even if some downplay the role of food, the real deal is that food is the biggest drug we take at least 3 times a day. Food can affect…

- her moods
- her skin
- her hair
- her sleep
- her thinking
- her energy

And it can affect her digestion.

The question of which came first, was it the Hashimoto's that affected her gut, or did her gut trigger her into Hashimoto's? I don't know the answer to that.

But, no matter which came first, you have to deal with

what's going on in the gut. And **the most power you both have in bringing healing to her is by choosing what she puts in her stomach.**

Finding and removing foods that trigger her reactions is one of the easiest ways to see if your woman is having a food reaction symptom (exhaustion, bloating, acid reflux, etc). Take away a food for 3-4 weeks, then add it back and see how she reacts. If she feels lousy or has odd symptoms, that's her body telling her what it doesn't like or tolerate well.

The main culprits when it comes to food sensitivities are... [3]

- Gluten
- Dairy
- Soy
- Grains (especially corn)
- Nightshades (like potatoes, tomatoes and peppers)
- Nuts and seeds

There are many ways to go about an <u>elimination diet</u>, and even tests that you can take to find out her inflammatory foods. Again, see the referenced articles and additional resources list for more to help you both choose the option that works best for her.

My Story:

When my wife, **Stacey**, was initially going through all her crazy symptoms, her stomach was one of the first things that went whacky. She just started not being able to eat the same things as she used to.

She was dealing with...

- **Exhaustion** – needing a nap for at least 2 hours after eating
- **Stomach problems** – running to the toilet just after eating a meal
- **Skin changes** – she'd get a hive like reaction on her face after eating
- **Heart palpitations** – not fun to have your heart freaking out
- **Asthmatic reactions** – gasping, burping, and full chest feeling
- **Anxiety** – certain foods would bring this on
- **Congestion** – especially after eating something she was reactive to (i.e. gluten)
- **Brain Fog** – yes, food would even make her thinking fuzzy
- **Dizziness** – where she would sit on the couch and wait for the world to stop spinning

This was before we realized that **foods with gluten (breads, pastas, donuts – basically anything with wheat, rye, or barley)** can cause a <u>lot</u> of problems for Hashi's people.

Now, my wife is Italian, and she did NOT want to give up her family foods – that would have been like giving up her childhood. But she was so tired of feeling like crap when she was eating it, that she finally agreed to try it.

Once we removed gluten from Stacey's diet, within about a week, she started noticing **her energy starting coming back** – which was super encouraging. Also, **her anxiety reduced by 50%!!!** (Yes, food can cause anxiety)

Because there is so much emotional reaction to giving up a whole food group, my wife Stacey addressed this in her book, **"You're Not Crazy, and You're Not Alone"** in her hilarious chapter, **"Fettucini Alfredo, Donut Holes, and other crimes of passion"**

Here's a portion of that chapter:

> "... I understand how it's more than letting go of gluten and dairy, corn and eggs, soy and nightshades and grains. It's about letting go of all the associations we make with food.
>
> I did all those other things on the list – I took care of my relationships, rest, supplements, meds, lifestyles, etc. They're all valuable and essential, but none of them can be a substitute for what the food changes provide.
>
> Myalgias went away, weight was lost, depression lifted, deeper sleep came, clarity of thinking returned and internal order resurfaced. I had no idea that cake was making me bitchy and that raw veggies made me want to have sex again. Who knew?
>
> I didn't know that my palpitations and racing heart were coming from food.
>
> That the anxiety I was feeling was coming from what I ate.
>
> That the heavy chest and labored breathing were from food sensitivities.
>
> That the tingling in my toes was from my menu choices. I had no idea the powerful role that food plays in our health... until I removed certain foods."

Removing gluten is truly one of the easiest shortcuts you can do <u>right now</u> to help her feel better.

I know, I know! – It's not an easy sell because there's gluten in just about everything worth eating! Stacey did the **buy every gluten free substitute on the market**, and actually ended up <u>gaining weight</u> and <u>feeling awful</u> for a while. She did best on a **whole food gluten free diet** – meats, vegetables, fruits, and some seeds.

The gluten free substitutes in the supermarket are definitely an option for those special occasions. But for her, she couldn't make those a part of her everyday diet.

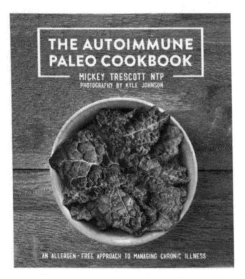

Our friend, and nutrition expert, **Mickey Trescott**, has a great recipe book out called **"<u>The Autoimmune Paleo Cookbook: An Allergen-Free Approach to Managing Chronic Illness</u>"**

Fortunately, this is a more common conversation these days than it was 20 years ago when Stacey was first diagnosed. Restaurants are getting on board too, so it's definitely doable. It just takes time and focus to get the gluten free foods that work for her.

But wait, there's more!

Some people take out gluten, and then feel amazingly better, but there are some that <u>only feel a little better</u>.

Gluten free may be just one piece of the puzzle. For my wife, she needed to also take out other foods - like eggs, dairy, nuts, and nightshades (potatoes, tomatoes, eggplant and peppers).

The important take-away here is – everyone is different. The more important take-away is – you can't give up, if one piece wasn't the whole puzzle. This is a process. She didn't get here overnight, so it's likely that it's not going to get fixed overnight.

Suggestions:

- **Watch for symptoms** - start noticing for any changes in symptoms within 15 minutes to an hour after her eating a meal

- **Remove offending foods** – using the <u>elimination diet</u>, remove a questionable food for 3-4 weeks, then add it back and see how she feels. It's quick, cheap, and relatively easy way to get clued into what works for her body

- **Use probiotics** – these can help restore the balance of good vs. bad stomach bacteria and help with digestion, help getting nutrients from food, and help balance the immune system

So, there you go, some science, our story, and some suggestions to get you started on healing your woman's stomach issues. Have her keep "listening" to what her body is saying works for her, and what doesn't.

The truth is, we all wish it were as easy as "take this pill, and you're fixed," but that is not the reality for many with Hashimoto's.

So, prepare yourself to go long, and keep working at it – together.

You guys can do it.

(Can't click on these? Well, this is just a book. Search online for the title, or go to **www.marriedtohashimotos.com/booklinks** for all of the links listed here, plus more.)

Referenced articles:

1. **What's Really Going On In Hashimoto's? Hashimoto's is more than just hypothyroidism**
   http://thyroidpharmacist.com/articles/whats-really-going-on-in-hashimotos

2. **Food Sensitivities And Hashimoto's - The Role of Food in Your Health Journey**
   http://thyroidpharmacist.com/articles/food-sensitivities-and-hashimotos

3. **The Gut-Thyroid Connection: 4 Steps for Breaking the Hashimoto's Autoimmune Cycle**
   http://avivaromm.com/gut-thyroid-connection

4. **Elimination Diet For Hashimoto's - Addressing Food Sensitivities in Hashimoto's**
   http://thyroidpharmacist.com/articles/elimination-diet-for-hashimotos

5. **The Thyroid-Gut Connection**
   https://chriskresser.com/the-thyroid-gut-connection

6. **How I inadvertently cut my Hashimoto's antibodies in half**
   http://hypothyroidmom.com/how-i-inadvertently-cut-my-hashimotos-antibodies-in-half

Additional resources:

The Gut and Autoimmune Thyroid Connection
http://thyroidpharmacist.com/articles/the-gut-and-autoimmune-thyroid-connection

Top 7 Hashimoto's Food Myths
http://thyroidpharmacist.com/articles/top-7-hashimotos-food-myths

Hashimoto's Diet Keys to Success
https://www.hashimotoshealing.com/hashimotos-diet-keys-to-success

Tight Junctions, Intestinal Permeability, and Autoimmunity: Celiac Disease and Type 1 Diabetes Paradigms
http://www.ncbi.nlm.nih.gov/pubmed/19538307

Incomplete Recovery and Individualized Responses of the Human Distal Gut Microbiota to Repeated Antibiotic Perturbation
http://www.pnas.org/content/early/2010/09/14/1000087107.full.pdf#page=1&view=FitH

What's up with her Moods?

Ok, guys... you ready for the chapter on roller coasters?
I mean... moods.

Buckle up, it's going to be a bumpy ride.

Ever felt hungry, tired, or achy? Maybe all three? Yeah, that's prolly going to affect your mood.

If it's true for you, it's especially true for your Hashi's woman.

Hashimoto's can affect her moods in serious ways.

Here's the science from **Cammi Balleck, Ph.D, CTN, ANCB Board Certified Naturopath:**

> "Our endocrine system is several glands that control all our hormones and neurotransmitters. Hormones and neurotransmitters are chemicals that control our mental and emotional states. These chemicals help the brain to balance emotions. When we have a problem with one gland such as the thyroid, all the other glands play into it as well. Our endocrine system works like a vehicle and all the parts have to be working at just the right time for us to feel good and be biochemically balanced." [1]

Also, in the early stages of Hashimoto's, the thyroid can sometimes swing to **hyperthyroid** (too much thyroid hormone) and back to **hypothyroid** (too little thyroid hormone) – that can cause some serious mood swings as well. [2]

There are even studies that link certain mental health issues to thyroid levels. [3]

So, it's highly likely that her mood swings are rooted in the medical reality of what she's going through.

Dang...

When I shared my article, **"Married to Hashimoto's: Where's the Woman I Married?"** over at **HypoThyroidmom.com**, I was surprised by how many women shared that their relationships had serious problems due to mood swings. Some relationships didn't make it through, or even realize it was Hashimoto's as the root of it.

What kinds of mood are we're talking about here?

- Depression
- Anger
- Anxiety
- Brain fog / fuzzy thinking
- Low sex drive

She may nag, and blow up smaller issues into bigger things.

Oh joy.

So for us guys, it's easy to focus on all these emotions, especially when they're directed <u>at</u> us.

I get that it's NOT fun to have a fire hose of emotion blasting you in the face – been there.

But for a minute let's get in her head and take in this all too familiar scenario...

- She's **not feeling well**. Her body is literally freaking out

- She's **gaining weight** and **feels like she's losing her old self**

- She **feels hopeless** and **out of control** when her doctor can't manage her thyroid level

- She **feels frustrated** when her doctor says her tests are finally "in range" but she still feels awful

- She's **not sleeping well**, and is awake for hours alone with her thoughts

- There's the **anxiety** of wondering, "Am I ever going to feel better again?"

- She feels **crazy**, when the doctors say this is an emotional issue and prescribe anti-anxiety, and anti-depression medication

- She is **misunderstood**, as an over-reacting hypochondriac

- She's **thought of as lazy** by family and friends because she looks "normal" on the outside

I hope that gives you the "other side" perspective.

It's gotta be like she's starring in her own movie where everything starts off fine. But then things change, and it's like she's in an alternate reality where her life slowly seems to go down the toilet no matter what she does.

Oh, and the movie doesn't end, for many women it goes on and on for <u>years</u>.

It's a nightmare to be thought of as a crazy, lazy, hypochondriac. It's no wonder than some of these women isolate themselves – many feel no one believes them anyway. Then there's the loneliness, thinking they're the only one going through this. Thankfully, there's a lot of online groups now of women who can relate.

As I'm writing this and looking back, I'm struck by what a jerk I was to my wife when she was first going through this. I really did not get how big an issue this was. I think most guys don't.

In the beginning, when there are just a few symptoms, it's very easy to dismiss.

"Ah, she's just being sensitive."

Even she may not know it's this tricky health issue.

Knowing what I know now, I want to hop into the nearest time machine, and go back to when this started (about 1996), and let her know she's not crazy. Then I'd help the younger me fast track her life back into a more healthy and happy future.

My Story:

When we're talking about moods and my wife – it's hard for me to look back and see which part was her being a passionate, Italian woman, and which parts were that her thyroid was going out of whack.

What I remember was that she started dealing with more fears and anxiety.

She did seem (to me) to be overly concerned with every new symptom. On my side, there was always something new going on for her to worry about.

- **My skin is freaking out**
- **I just can't lose weight**
- **My hair on my legs just isn't growing**
- **Why do I keep getting infections?**
- **Does this skin issue look normal to you?**
- **What do you think is going on?**
- **I'm having a reaction to this food! I can't eat this**
- **That spray cleaner is making me sick**
- **Good god, why am I using the bathroom so often?**
- **What did you say? I can't even think clearly**

All of this adds to her fear, frustration, aches and pains.

And if I wasn't being understanding enough, or paying enough attention, it was easy for me to be the anger lightning rod.

This was really hard, because I love my wife, and yet sometimes she's taking her anger and frustration out on me. Some of it was justified and some wasn't. So, when I'd try to comfort her, **sometime it felt like I was trying hug a porcupine.**

At home during these times, it wasn't a lot of fun. I'd go to work, and it ended up being a more peaceful place – there was order and I got appreciated for the work I did. But work and home are not the same, obviously.

My wife is my life partner. She just wants to feel protected, safe, and loved. I have my own version of that – I want to share my life and resources with someone who loves me and shows appreciation for what I'm doing. No one wants a life that's a constant grind.

But our reality then was that life was not fun. Her health was the big issue taking over... everything. Without her health, we didn't get to fully enjoy the fun times.

When you don't know that these crazy moods are part of medical condition, it's easy to think she's just being a crank. So sometimes I was in that helpful zone, and other times I just got frustrated and angry with her.

I know that for me, my issue was that I didn't want to have to deal with ANY health issues. My mom had died in her late 40s from lung cancer, so when it came to health conversations, my brain really wanted to check out. Plus life was already busy with work, family, kids, and other commitments.

So, I left her to figure it out essentially alone. I mean, I took her to doctor appointments, and was there in the room, but I often wasn't paying attention.

What she needed was a consistent partner in this. Someone to talk with her about her concerns and fears - which doctor was good or not, what the most recent tests said; and sometime she just needed to not talk about anything and just be held.

My advice to the younger me, don't give yourself such a hard time. I didn't know what was going on, and when I did realize, years had already passed. You can't do anything about that time.

But you can pick up the ball, and take it from <u>here</u>. Leave the guilt behind. Make amends if you need to.

There was no Guys' Guide to Hashimoto's on this disease 20 years ago. Now there's TONS of information, but it's overkill to Google Hashimoto's. It's mostly geared towards women (understandable as women are affected much more than men), or it's DEEP medical research that makes your eyes glaze over when you read it.

Heck, that's why I put this together.

OK, now back to our story.

What's really interesting is that Hashimoto's women have a general profile. In their strength, they're uber-productive, caring, and dynamic. The flip side of that is there can be issues of trust, self-rejection, fear, perfectionism, control, and guilt. So add all of that mental baggage to her physical symptoms, and it's not hard to see why her moods could be over the top.

Now, let's take a look at some practical things you can do now to help her, and help you keep sane.

Things that can help her mood...

- **Less stress** – another Captain Obvious moment here. This is probably one of the most important steps toward her health. The chemicals that stress releases in the body aren't good for healthy people, but they're especially bad for someone with a compromised immune system.

- **Talk to her** – or maybe I should have written **listen to her**. Heck, do both. Part of what will help relieve stress for her, is to be known. This can be as simple as taking a walk together around the block, or someplace she finds restful – like the beach, or a park. Then just throw out the bait,

"Hon, how are you doing today?"

BOOM!

It's likely the barrage of words to follow will cover a LOT of ground. I have found that it doesn't even matter if we figure something out, or get to the bottom of everything. What matters is us as men checking in on our women and keep the communication going.
You need to be heard too.

- **Removing foods that jack up her body** – I address this in the "**What's up with Her Stomach?**" section. If there are foods that she's sensitive to, you bet it's going to affect her mood too.

116

- **Sex** – Yep, had to put this in there. What?! Sex is a mood enhancer - and there definitely is science to back me up on this. See the **"What the Heck Happened to Our Sex Life?"** section for more.

- **Yoga** – gentle yoga like **yin, hatha, or kundalini yoga,** not the aggressive or strenuous kind. Since her stress needs to be reduced, this is a great way for her to regularly be mindful and relax. [4]

- **Supplements** – Being depleted in proper nutrition absolutely can affect her moods. So, supplements can really help here.

- **The right medicines** - If her doctor is only looking at and treating her individual symptoms, and still feels awful, it's likely time to see someone new. Depression and anxiety's root cause is not a lack of drugs. You need to find a trusted medicine practitioner to help you – people who are going to look at the big picture. Some women suffer on the "standard" Hashimoto's treatment unnecessarily. See the **"Conventional vs. Alternative – What's the Deal?"** section for more.

How to help her with this...

The first order of business (if you haven't done it already)...

- **Acknowledge that her symptoms are because of a legit medical issue**

- **Apologize** (Wait... what? If you need to. Not sure? Ask her.)

The goal is to get on the same page, so as a team you can move on to the important next steps for her health.
If you've been minimizing her symptoms, and treating her poorly, that has <u>got</u> to be addressed.

Would you want to partner with someone who didn't believe in you?

<u>Important side note</u>: what I laid out above is what my wife, Stacey, and I went through.

It's the inspiration for the book that she wrote, **"You're Not Crazy and You're Not Alone"** –

I highly recommend it.

No other book out there is addressing the mental game of Hashimoto's and how important it is to her healing.

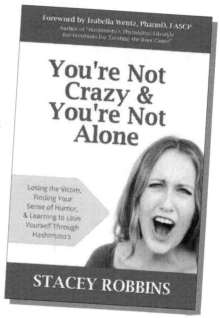

Want to be a hero? Get a copy for her.

If you go to **staceyrobbins.com** and sign up for her mailing list, she'll send you the top 2 chapters from the book for free. See if she likes what's she's reading.

You can also read Stacey's powerful article, **The Power of "I Believe"** over at **staceyrobbins.com** too – just search for it online.

Hang in there. It really is possible to get her health and emotions stabilized again.

It may not be without bumps along the road, but it is very doable.

(Can't click on these? Well, this is just a book. Search online for the title, or go to **www.marriedtohashimotos.com/booklinks** for all of the links listed here, plus more.)

Referenced articles:

1. **Anxiety? Panic Attacks? Depression? Mood Swings? The Thyroid Roller Coaster Ride**
   http://hypothyroidmom.com/anxiety-panic-attacks-depression-mood-swings-the-thyroid-roller-coaster-ride

2. **Hashimoto's Thyroiditis: We Can Win This Battle!**
   http://www.huffingtonpost.com/dr-raphael-kellman/hashimotos-thyroiditis-we_2_b_7118690.html

3. **Thyroid and Mental Health Articles**
   http://www.stopthethyroidmadness.com/thyroid-depression-mental-health/articles

4. **Can Doing Yoga Improve Thyroid Health?**
   http://www.naturalendocrinesolutions.com/articles/can-doing-yoga-improve-thyroid-health

Related links:

- **Thyroid Disease: Can It Affect a Person's Mood?**
  http://www.mayoclinic.org/thyroid-disease/expert-answers/faq-20058228

- **How Adrenals Can Wreak Havoc – Symptoms of Low Cortisol**
  http://www.stopthethyroidmadness.com/adrenal-info/symptoms-low-cortisol

What's up with her Energy?

One of the many symptoms she may have with Hashimoto's is low energy.

Ok, that first statement is a major *under*statement.

If I had a dollar for every Hashimoto's woman who said that she wakes up tired, goes all day exhausted, and then climbs in bed, only to be awake for hours with insomnia, and **finally** falls asleep – only to do it all over again – I'd be a very, very rich man.

Since the thyroid is referred to as the thermostat of the body when it comes to metabolism (converting the food you eat into available energy), it's not surprising that one of the biggest symptoms Hashimoto's women deal with is low energy. They feel exhausted, and drag around like a zombie even after enough sleep. Yet another symptom of the body thermostat being off is her complaining of cold hands and feet. [1]

One of the biggest commodities we have in life is our energy – it's the currency that allows us to invest in our goals and our dreams. But if you wake up after a full night's sleep, yet don't have the energy to get out of bed, how are you going to make those dreams happen?

Here's the good news, there's something you can do about it.

Before we get to the suggestions, let's do a flyby on the science.

The Science:

The simple version, we get our energy from the food we eat. I like this description from **livestrong.com**:

> "Whether you are asleep, awake, exercising or reclining on your couch, your cells require a constant source of energy to carry on their metabolic tasks. The jobs of enzymes, structural proteins, hormones, fatty acids and other important molecules continue around the clock, as do the processes of cellular repair, regeneration and reproduction. Your body gets its needed energy from foods, which are all ultimately funneled into cellular 'furnaces' called mitochondria, where nutrients are converted to high-energy molecules called adenosine triphosphate, or ATP." [2]

So, food gets converted into energy. Check out the chapter **"What's Going on with Her Stomach?"** to understand why healing her gut is a huge priority.

My Story:

Back before my wife was diagnosed with Hashimoto's, her hands, feet, and well, her butt was often colder than other parts of her body – classic low thyroid symptoms. It was a running joke for us when we were first married. Looking back on that now – not quite so funny, as I had no clue it was related to Hashimoto's.

Her body was giving clues as to what was going on, if only I had been paying closer attention.

Stacey had her own businesses, so she'd work from 6am in the morning until late at night. And the next morning she'd be exhausted.

Her eyes felt gritty, her body was in pain, and she took forever to wake up.

I want to remind you, she was 25 at the time, and she was a morning person <u>and</u> a night owl who could function really well on very little sleep. But that changed after being hit in 2 car accidents, our stressful marriage, and her father dying unexpectedly. She was a different person.

I remember her trying to describe to me the level of fatigue she was feeling. She would say, **"It's like the bones of my soul are tired."**

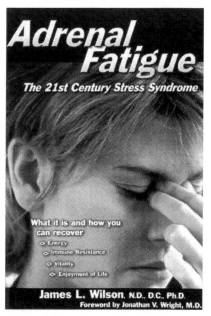

10 years, 2 kids, and a cross-country move later... the exhaustion went to a whole new level. That's when we learned about **adrenal fatigue**.

What's Adrenal Fatigue?

It's a bedfellow to Hashimoto's, and can happen after a shock, trauma, accident, injury, surgery, or after a *freaking lifetime of chronic stress*.

123

It's when the part of your body that helps you manage fight or flight, gets used up. And instead of being able to function under stressful situations, you have profound fatigue instead. The adrenals are like the brake pads for the stressful parts of your life. When they get worn out, there's a lot of screeching involved.

One of the books that really made a difference with this was, **Adrenal Fatigue: The 21st Century Stress Syndrome** by **James Wilson**

The good things you're doing to help her thyroid can also help with her adrenal fatigue.

According to Dr. Wilson:

"Adrenal fatigue (hypoadrenia) is a collection of signs and symptoms, known as a syndrome, that results when the adrenal glands function below the necessary level. Most commonly associated with intense or prolonged stress, it can also arise during or after acute or chronic infections, especially respiratory infections such as influenza, bronchitis or pneumonia. As the name suggests, its paramount symptom is **fatigue that is not relieved by sleep**."

"Most medical doctors are not aware of adrenal fatigue. They only recognize Addison's disease, which is the most extreme end of low adrenal function. Astute doctors who are familiar with the varying degrees of decreased adrenal function usually test the adrenal hormone levels in the saliva." [3]

So, in addition to a gluten-free diet, proper hydration, supplements, and thyroid meds, the adrenal component helped us to make lifestyle changes for my wife.

Changes like:

- Bed before 10pm (aim for 8-9 hours of sleep)
- No alarm clocks
- Peaceful lighting
- Peaceful sounds / music
- Yoga (the gentle / restorative kind)
- Meditation
- "Legs up the wall" (a yoga pose)
- Grounding, a.k.a. Earthing (getting out in nature)
- No alcohol (or less of it)
- Eating every 2½ to 3 hours
- Dandelion tea
- Removing toxic relationships (just ask her, she knows who)
- Cutting back on work hours or switching jobs

<u>Suggestions</u>:

Address these energy-stealing issues... [4,5]

- **Getting enough sleep** – Captain Obvious here. Start with the basics and see if that helps. If she gets a good night's sleep (shoot for 8-9 hours) and wakes up happily and singing, you may have found part of the solution.

- **Low TSH** – the main symptom of low TSH (Thyroid Stimulating Hormone) is low energy. The appropriate level of TSH is a very important for proper energy and function of the body. Work with your doctor or practitioner here to regulate her TSH level to the level that works for her.

The main issue you'll run into here is that most TSH blood tests have outdated TSH reference levels – meaning your woman with Hashimoto's can have a TSH level that is "in range" and still feel awful. See the "**Conventional vs. Alternative – What's the Deal?**" section for more about the standard TSH level, which is a point of controversy and see what the new proposed TSH level should be.

- **Anemia** – is low iron and another reason for low energy. You can determine this through a blood test.

- **Food sensitivity** – she may find that certain foods just leave her wiped out. The common culprits are gluten, dairy, soy, nuts, eggs, nightshades, and corn. See the chapter "**What's Going on with Her Stomach?**"

- **Low blood sugar** – after eating a carb heavy meal – or waiting too long in-between meals – her energy can really drop. Have her try adding more protein and fats with her meals to even out blood sugar issues.

- **Get the gut in order** – since the digestion is a hugely important place where we get our energy from. Again, see the chapter "**What's Going on with Her Stomach?**"

- **Gentle exercise instead of hard exercise** – If she's finding herself unusually wiped out after exercise, she may need to lighten up for a while. It's about listening to her body to see what works for her. See the **Exercise Intolerance** article listed in the referenced articles section.

- **Add vitamin B12** – known as the "energy nutrient" bodies need to do our basic essential functions. Some women need different types of B-12 because of Methylation issues, see the referenced articles section.

- **Get out in the sun** – a simple thing to do that can help Hashi's people feel better and more energetic. Skip the sunglasses and have her take in the midday sun – take a walk, read in the park, have a picnic. You get the idea.

Here's the good news. Depending on what your woman is dealing with, sometimes energy can increase in a matter of days. When my wife took gluten out of her diet, she ended up having energy within a week. We she went on a full on elimination diet, she was a different person in **30** days.

With proper supplementation, and meds, and a properly regulated thyroid, she was almost like super women. These things all work in concert with each other.

Everyone's right treatment is different, but the bottom line is, put your energy here, so that she can get her energy back.

(Can't click on these? Well, this is just a book. Search online for the title, or go to **www.marriedtohashimotos.com/booklinks** for all of the links listed here, plus more.)

Referenced articles:

1. **Thyroid and Cold Intolerance!**
   http://thyroidpharmacist.com/articles/thyroid-and-cold-intolerance

2. **How Does the Body Change Food Into Energy?**
   http://www.livestrong.com/article/496198-how-does-our-body-change-food-into-energy-we-can-use

3. **FAQ on Adrenal Fatigue**
   https://adrenalfatigue.org/faq-on-adrenal-fatique

4. **Top 10 Tips for Overcoming Hashimoto's Fatigue**
   http://thyroidpharmacist.com/articles/top-10-tips-for-overcoming-hashimotos-fatigue

5. **10 Ways to Overcome Fatigue with a Low Thyroid**
   http://hypothyroidmom.com/10-ways-to-overcome-fatigue-with-a-low-thyroid

Related links:

Finding the Balance: The Story of Exercise Intolerance
http://www.thyroidchange.org/our-blog/finding-the-balance-the-story-of-exercise-intolerance

The Connection: Vitamin B12, Methylation and Thyroid Symptoms
http://www.hashimotosawareness.org/the-connection-vitamin-b12-methylation-and-thyroid-symptoms

What's up with her Weight?

Ok, are we really going there? Normally this is the "I won't touch this with a ten-foot pole" area.

It's ok, you don't have to read this to her. It's just for you, ok? Whew.

So, yeah. I'd like to say that women dealing with Hashimoto's didn't have to deal with weight issues, but that would not be true. Some actually have a hard time putting weight on – but that's not the norm – more often than not, you'll hear about women gaining weight.

If you're like me, your wife has been slowly, or not so slowly, increasing in size and trying really hard not to. She's tried everything to pare down including exercise, dieting, Spanx, etc. – not really knowing what's going on in her body, and trying to use old methods to deal with the new health situation. At some point, the Hashimoto's diagnosis comes, and we all realize what's been going on is a complicated hypothyroid autoimmune issue.

What the heck do we do now?

I immediately think...

First, I want her to be healthy.

And second, I'd love for her to be back to a healthy weight.

Not the weirdo Barbie doll weight, but the version where she's comfortable in her own skin. Ok, well maybe that's a whole different topic and therapy session. But, you know what I mean.

Here's our before Hashimoto's and after Hashimoto's diagnosis photo of my wife at her highest weight...

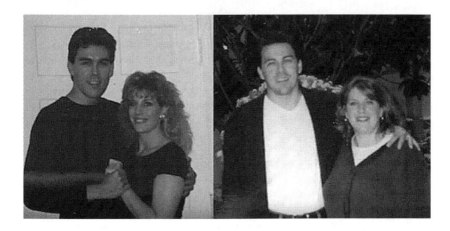

Yeah, it's like there was no stopping the weight gain. At her highest, she tipped the scales at 270.

I'm pretty sure I gained some sympathy weight too.

(Don't worry, we share this all over the place now, she's cool with me sharing that)

So, in case you didn't you realize by now, **weight gain is part of the hypothyroid / Hashimoto's most common symptoms**.

Oh joy.

Of course, our next stop is the flyby on the science.

The Science

When it comes to why Hashimoto's patient have weight issues, there are some main players.

Her Thyroid Levels

First off, weight gain is right up there in the top most common Hashimoto's symptoms[1], which makes sense since **the thyroid's main job is to control metabolism,** which is our body's ability to break down food and convert it to energy.[2]

top 10 symptoms

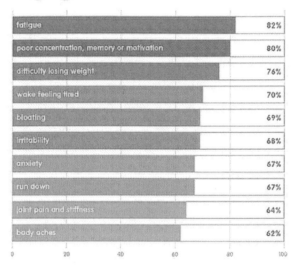

fatigue	82%
poor concentration, memory or motivation	80%
difficulty losing weight	76%
wake feeling tired	70%
bloating	69%
irritability	68%
anxiety	67%
run down	67%
joint pain and stiffness	64%
body aches	62%

Hashimoto's Symptom Survey from nearly 3,000 participants
Source: hypothyroidmom.com

I'm going to try to keep it simple here and just address the pertinent parts. The thyroid gland creates the hormone T4, the *inactive* form.

Next important step is that the liver converts the T4 into T3, the *active* form.

T3 is where the magic happens. The cells in our bodies really respond to T3.

Dr. Joseph Mercola addresses this part best:

"If everything is working properly, you will make what you need and have the correct amounts of T3 and T4, which control the metabolism of every cell in your body.

If your T3 is inadequate, either by scarce production or not converting properly from T4, your whole system suffers.

T3 is critically important because it tells the nucleus of your cells to send messages to your DNA to rev up your metabolism by burning fat. This is how T3 lowers cholesterol levels, regrows hair, and **helps keep you lean."** [2]

So, here's another tricky part – if her thyroid level is low, the old standard **"just eat less, and move your body more"** formula likely won't work for weight loss. If you're woman is frustrated because she's dieting, and exercising like crazy, but it isn't making a difference, this one of the main reasons why.

Her Food

Ok guys, next up is food. The bummer news is – it's complicated.

Why not just diet?

Diet becomes a 4-letter word if she's eating the wrong type of food. She can be actually contributing to the inflammation that is already part of the problem with Hashimoto's. Because less food isn't the answer when you have a body that is enflamed by certain foods.

Plus, her digestion may already be slow anyway. So, pulling out a diet bar, a low calorie drink, or a frozen meal for weight loss likely isn't going to help. If she's already tried that, it's time to try something new.

Here's what **Dr. Josh Axe** says:

> "Hypothyroidism can have a negative effect beginning in the stomach. When thyroid hormone production and/or absorption is low, this restricts the stomach's ability to manufacture a hormone called gastrin. Gastrin is responsible for the production of hydrochloric acid, also known as stomach acid.
>
> Having sufficient stomach acid is crucial to our digestion. When food is not broken down well enough, this can cause the small intestine to not allow it to pass. In essence, the food can stagnate and begin to rot in the stomach producing symptoms of heartburn.
>
> This lack of stomach acid can also cause impaired absorption of vital nutrients including vitamin B12, iron, and calcium. When this occurs, anemias can develop as a result of the underlying hypothyroidism."[3]

So, what does that mean?

The goal isn't just to lose weight.

The goal is to get her health back to a stable place where it can function optimally, which includes losing weight.

It's up to you guys to find the right foods for her to eat.

This is when I wish a pill would take care of everything – truly. My wife's experience with finding the right food (which you'll read about next) came after trying the "medication only" route. But when your woman is feeling awful, and the doctors are scratching their heads, you get more willing to try things outside of the box of what standard medicine offers. And heck, if what the doctors were offering worked, we would have stopped there.

> **"The food you eat can be either the safest and most powerful form of medicine or the slowest form of poison."**— Ann Wigmore

Most people resist changing their food. I know I do.

For years I ate whatever I wanted (you know, when I was indestructible). And then I started noticing as I got older that I would get congested after some foods, or be wiped out after some meals.

Food is powerful, and for your woman to feel better and be able to lose weight, it's absolutely worth the effort to find what foods work for her.

Here's the thing you need to know up front – there are likely foods that are not good for her, maybe temporarily, maybe

134

forever – I don't know. After the elimination diet of removing, and re-adding some, she'll know which ones those are. If it's a temptation to eat foods that don't work for her, remind her of how poorly she felt eating it, and how good she feels without it.

Now, there are some diets out there that Hashimoto's women have found helpful. There are others, but these are the top ones.

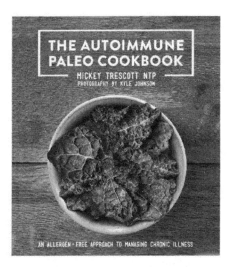

- **Paleo Diet**
- **Autoimmune Paleo Diet**
- **Vegan Autoimmune Paleo Diet**
- **Specific Carbohydrate Diet (SCD)**
- **Body Ecology Diet**

Our friend, and Nutritional Therapy Practitioner, **Mickey Trescott**, wrote the **Autoimmune Paleo Cookbook**.

Stacey's made some of the recipes from there, and our family just loves them.

Leaky Gut

There is another stomach condition, known as **Leaky Gut**. It's not medically recognized... yet. **TIME magazine has affirmed the science**[4], and the traditional medical community is coming around. Many of the main players in Hashimoto's treatments have already being working with this for quite a while, and many frustrated and sick people have benefitted from following the protocol.

What's special about this condition is that it can address the autoimmune response our stomach has to food – that's something very pertinent for Hashimoto's patients because Hashimoto's is an autoimmune disease.

Let's read more of what **Dr. Josh Axe** has to say...

> "When someone has **leaky gut** (often referred to as **increased intestinal permeability**), the "net" in your digestive tract gets damaged, which causes even bigger holes to develop in your net, so things that normally can't pass through, are now be able to. Some of the things that can now pass through include proteins like gluten, bad bacteria and undigested foods particles. Toxic waste can also leak from the inside of your intestinal wall into your bloodstream causing an immune reaction" [5]

These particles end up going where they are <u>not</u> supposed to be and rouse the body's immune system to attack these food particles – and that causes serious inflammation in the stomach. It's very important to heal that inflammation in the stomach first which helps put out the autoimmune "fire" that is raging.

Here are some of the possible Leaky Gut symptoms... [5]

- **Bloating**
- **Food sensitivities**
- **Fatigue**
- **Joint pain**
- **Headaches**

- **Skin issues like rosacea and acne**
- **Digestive problems**
- **Weight gain**

If you can get her gut better, it could drastically improve her health.

I look at this like an extra specialized tool in my toolbox (and I love having extra tools) – and if she needs this tool, it can be a life saver.

There's a pretty amazing video interview of a New York Times reporter, **Susannah Meadows,** [6] (a trained sceptic) and how she dealt with one of her children having serious stomach problems. She believes the Leaky Gut protocol helped her son. She wrote about it all in her New York Times article[7] as well.

You want to take time to see the interview – quite amazing.

One diet that specifically addresses Leaky Gut is called **the GAPS diet,** there are other variations. See the referenced link section.

Stress / Adrenal Fatigue / Cortisol

Let's start with this from **mayoclinic.org**:

> "When you encounter a perceived threat — a large dog barks at you during your morning walk, for instance — your hypothalamus, a tiny region at the base of your brain, sets off an alarm system in your body. Through a combination of nerve and hormonal signals, this system prompts your adrenal glands, located atop your kidneys, to release a surge of

hormones, including adrenaline and cortisol. Adrenaline increases your heart rate, elevates your blood pressure and boosts energy supplies. Cortisol, the primary stress hormone, increases sugars (glucose) in the bloodstream, enhances your brain's use of glucose and increases the availability of substances that repair tissues.

Cortisol also curbs functions that would be nonessential or detrimental in a fight-or-flight situation. It alters immune system responses and suppresses the digestive system, the reproductive system and growth processes. This complex natural alarm system also communicates with regions of your brain that control mood, motivation and fear." [8]

Many Hashi women have experienced prolonged periods of stress. It could have been in her childhood, her teen years, or adulthood. It may even have been throughout her whole life. Imagine living like you're always being chased by a bear. How could you not be exhausted? How could your body not be affected? How could you not feel hopeless? This is bad for her as her body isn't designed to live in the red line area most of the time. I addressed also in the **Adrenal Fatigue** section of the **"What's up with her energy?"** chapter.

Here's the big takeaway you need to know – **if she's really stressed out, it's going to make it harder for her to lose weight.**

Arrrggh!!

Yep, the relevant symptom here is "decreased metabolism"... *again.*

Oh, and if that wasn't enough, **long term stress / cortisol lowers her thyroid hormones.** [9]

Sheesh!

So, what's the prescription? If you want your woman to have more energy, and be able to lose weight effectively - lowering her stress <u>has</u> to be part of the action plan.

<u>My Story</u>

My girl, back in the day, was something to behold. Young, trim, sexy, talented, funny – she was a catch, for sure. I was a handsome guy too (hopefully I still am).

We dated, played, worked, married, traveled, and more. I'm compressing a lot, but there was a lot of life going on before Hashimoto's hit our life and drastically changed my wife's health 7 years into our marriage. We were in our late twenties when the fit hit the shan.

For the weight part of my story, I need to share about what we were like back then.

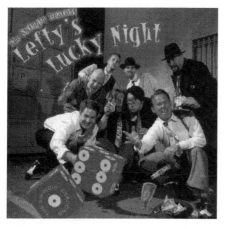

Now me, I was a pretty easy going guy (still am). I was a musician, and was playing different gigs in bands all over Southern California. I sang and played saxophone in various pop, rock, jazz and swing bands. Very fun to get dressed up and play a lively gig. Oh, and you got paid too. Booyah!

So, I would gather up my saxes, and take along my svelte wife to some cool club and we'd play, drink, and have a fun time with the band and other audience revelers.

We were this couple that, forgive the pun, made beautiful music together. Stacey was a singer, and a piano player too. Together we played clubs, restaurants, corporate events, private parties, and more weddings than I can count.

We had the whole package – an attractive talented couple using our talents and having a ball. She also taught music lessons, kids choirs, musical camps. Truly, I'm making this list and I'm amazed at all she managed.

All the while Stacey was helping me get my act together. Aside from helping me in my business dealings (she was really talented that way), at some point she saved enough to get me a Selmer Mark VI saxophone. That's a not only a professional saxophone, it's one of a few made in France in the 1960's that were just amazing sounding. Pro players still look for these today. That's the kind of person my wife is – very generous.

Then, things started to change for Stacey. She started gaining weight, and not feeling well.

She's no slouch, she tried to push through, but that's a recipe for burnout when you have Hashimoto's.

She also had the stress of her dad dying, we were having marital problems, and she got hit in 2 separate different car accidents.

It was not a happy time.

Plus her thyroid was swelling (that's called goiter) and it was pushing into her esophagus and making her choke when she ate. She was trying to hide what she was going through by chewing her food 40+ times for each bite.

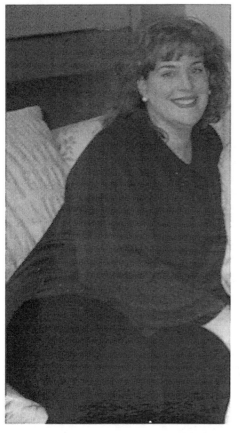

So, at the end of it of all this madness, I had a sick, depressed, low energy, fat wife.

She didn't feel good about herself – moping around in dark clothing and trying to hide her body. And people treated her differently – family, friend, and strangers.

She reached a point where she couldn't handle the stress anymore, she couldn't push through.

I remember that we were driving back from Las Vegas over Thanksgiving. Stacey was coughing and choking from on some food she was eating.

And me, I was *pissed*.

I was tired of all these symptoms and her anxiety at... everything. The inconvenience – all this health stuff was cramping my style and was really not fun.

So, we pulled over on the side of the desert road, I think I was irritated at Stacey for choking on her food. She was crying and confessed that she was having all these crazy symptoms, and couldn't handle the stress anymore.

What Did I Do?

Well, I would like to say I was this awesome husband who put his frustration aside, swooped in, comforted, and took care of her. But I was mixed bag – I cared about her, and I was selfish.

Instead of "for better or for worse", I was more like a "for better or for as long as it doesn't take too long."

I told her, "Why didn't you tell me? We need to get you to a doctor."

Stacey instinctively stopped eating solid food for a about a month – it was too stressful for her.

Then we went to see a surgeon about removing Stacey's thyroid.

Now, that is NOT a small deal for singer; one possible side effect could have been that the surgery could nick her vocal cord nerve – paralyzing her voice.

The surgeon was cautious about taking out her thyroid, and asked if she could go three months without solid food. So, we blended all her foods, tried to craft a peaceful life, and started slow, but steady exercise – as in only 5 minutes of slow walking a day. As she felt better we slowly increased the walking time.

By the time we got to our new doctor, Stacey's goiter had shrunk and her thyroid was almost back to a normal size. Oh, and she was **70 pounds lighter.**

Suggestions

- **Understand what she's going through.**

  You're already doing your part by reading this book, but also have your wife read this powerful article by my wife Stacey – **It's a "Beautiful" Thing.** It's over at **hypothyroidmom.com** [10]

  P.S. you should read this too.

- **Prioritize a healthy gut over a skinny body.**

  Work with a like-minded health practitioner to help guide her to a health gut and body.

- **Encourage her to take care of herself, even if she's at a weight she doesn't like.**

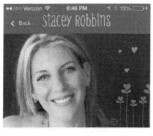

This is your life. If you love the script, keep going.

Stacey Robbins is an author and speaker who inspires

My wife has two very encouraging products for women, her **Iphone app Bloom Beautiful** and her book, **Bloom Beautiful: Inspirational Musings and Memes.**

One of her quotes says...

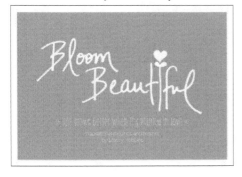

"Love is a wonderful inspiration, but it's a terrible reward"

What does that mean?

It means that if you are holding back part of yourself, or your care for your woman for when she loses weight, you are training her that she's worth less at a higher weight, and worth more when she's thinner.

So, encourage your wife to put on that cute outfit, put on her make-up, do her hair, and treat herself like she's worth taking care of <u>now</u> – because she is.

- **Love and value her now.**

  Remember, this time is hopefully temporary. There are lessons for you during this uncomfortable time.

  Don't miss it.

  When she's thinner and healthier, and on her game again, she will really trust that your love is the real deal <u>because you loved her during this "not beautiful" time</u>.

If you are rejecting of her when she's heavy, and then you're connected to her when she's thin, you haven't earned her trust, because you're only loving her conditionally.

But if you love her <u>through</u> this time, then she will trust you when she <u>gets through</u> this time.

(Can't click on these? Well, this is just a book. Search online for the title, or go to **www.marriedtohashimotos.com/booklinks** for all of the links listed here, plus more.)

Referenced articles:

1. **The Cold-Hard Truth About Hashimoto's Symptoms**
   http://hypothyroidmom.com/the-cold-hard-truth-about-hashimotos-symptoms

2. **What You Need to Know About Your Thyroid Health**
   http://articles.mercola.com/thyroid.aspx

3. **Thyroid Disease & Digestive Problems**
   http://www.totalhealthmagazine.com/Thyroid-Health/Thyroid-Disease-Digestive-Problems.html

4. **You Asked: Is Leaky Gut Syndrome a Real Thing? (The latest science says yes...)**
   http://time.com/4178015/leaky-gut-syndrome-probiotics

5. **4 Steps to Heal Leaky Gut and Autoimmune Disease**
   https://draxe.com/4-steps-to-heal-leaky-gut-and-autoimmune-disease

6. **(VIDEO STORY: New York Times Reporter) Could Leaky Gut Be What's Troubling You?**
   http://www.doctoroz.com/article/could-leaky-gut-be-troubling-you

7. **(New York Times Reporter Story) The Boy With a Thorn in His Joints**
   http://www.nytimes.com/2013/02/03/magazine/the-boy-with-a-thorn-in-his-joints.html

8. **Chronic Stress Puts Your Health at Risk**
   http://www.mayoclinic.org/healthy-lifestyle/stress-management/in-depth/stress/art-20046037

9. **Cortisol and Thyroid Hormones**
   http://hypothyroidmom.com/cortisol-and-thyroid-hormones

10. **It's a 'Beautiful' Thing... (by Stacey Robbins)**
    http://hypothyroidmom.com/its-a-beautiful-thing

Related links:

- **Weight Loss and Hypothyroidism:**
  Quite the Odd Couple
  http://hypothyroidmom.com/weight-loss-and-hypothyroidism-quite-the-odd-couple

- **Hashimoto's Diet: Keys to Success**
  https://www.hashimotoshealing.com/hashimotos-diet-keys-to-success

- **Eating with Hashimoto's Disease**
  http://thescienceofeating.com/food-combining-how-it-works/eating-with-hashimotos-disease

- **Stomach Acid – the Why and the What**
  http://www.stopthethyroidmadness.com/stomach-acid

Gut health links:

- **Leaky Gut: The missing piece in many Autoimmune Diseases, like Hashimoto's Thyroiditis**
  http://hypothyroidmom.com/leaky-gut-the-missing-piece-in-many-autoimmune-diseases-like-hashimotos-thyroiditis

- **How I Reversed Hashimoto's (a Thyroid Autoimmune) Disease with Food**
  http://deliciouslyorganic.net/reverse-hashimotos-thyroid-disease

- **Autoimmune Gut-Repair Diet**
  https://drknews.com/autoimmune-gut-repair-diet

Leaky Gut:

- **4 Steps to Heal Leaky Gut and Autoimmune Disease**
  https://draxe.com/4-steps-to-heal-leaky-gut-and-autoimmune-disease

- **Leaky Gut Syndrome in Plain English – and How to Fix It**
  http://scdlifestyle.com/2010/03/the-scd-diet-and-leaky-gut-syndrome

- **GAPS Diet: Heal Your Autoimmune Disease Now**
  http://www.thehealthyhomeeconomist.com/heal-your-autoimmune-disease-now

- **What Is A Leaky Gut? (And How Can It Cause So Many Health Issues?)**
  http://www.thepaleomom.com/2012/03/what-is-leaky-gut-and-how-can-it-cause.html

Stress / Adrenal Fatigue / Cortisol:

- **Cortisol and Thyroid Hormones**
  http://hypothyroidmom.com/cortisol-and-thyroid-hormones

- **Are Your Adrenals Sabotaging Your Health?**
  http://thyroidpharmacist.com/articles/are-your-adrenals-sabotaging-your-health

Hashimoto's, Health, and Happiness:

- **Stacey Robbins** (That would be my wife)
  http://staceyrobbins.com

What the Heck Happened to Our Sex Life?

Ah... sex. Such a wonderful gift to humanity.

We love it. When it's available, it's like manna from heaven.

If we're starved for it, the lack of it can be its own special hell.

Of course, you can take care of business yourself, but that's not really the same, is it?

We crave physical contact with another.

And when we're firing on all cylinders, it becomes more than sex. It's a partnership – we share life's amazing moments, mundane moments, and even painful moments.

Sex with that special person is much more than just the physical act, it becomes intimacy. It can be physical, mental, and spiritual.

Ah...

Um... Is that too poetic?

Oh man, I went off on a tangent there, didn't I?

Ahem...

Truth be told, sometimes we just want sex, for the release of having sex. It's such a natural stress reliever, aside from feeling amazing.

Ok, but what if your partner, who's going through Hashimoto's,

doesn't

want

sex.

And I don't mean, "Hmmm... maybe I could be interested now, or maybe not".

I mean, she feels totally – *nothing*.

No desire, or barely there desire.

And she likely has no idea why the desire isn't there.

All she knows is that she just doesn't feel like it.

I know – most guys can't relate to that at all.
We are usually "ready" just about any time.

Try this on for perspective:

Have you ever been so sick from the flu that you threw up everything? You know what I mean. And then, when you were done with that, you clean up and walk back out into the living room, a bit dazed, and all you want to do is lie on the couch... forever.

Next, your lovely woman sees you, and brings out your favorite meal – a bacon double cheeseburger, with fries and a beer. I mean, it's <u>exactly</u> how you'd want it...

IF you were feeling well.

But right now...

You absolutely have NO desire to eat.
ZERO.

You can't even imagine it. Even though it's your favorite.

Normally you can eat that all day long, every day.

Of course, you know what's going on – your body is taking care of other important issues right now, and it makes you not hungry for a very valid reason. You may not eat much for days while you're recovering.

She protests, **"How could you not want this? I made it especially for you. You always love this. I can't believe you're doing this to me.**

Don't you *care* about me?"

How's that for perspective?

Now, that's not a perfect example, because unlike you with the flu, most women don't realize that it's their thyroid or adrenals that are at the root of their lack of sex drive – and the husbands usually don't know either.

Now let's get back to the issue at hand: sex.

You take that important element out of the relationship, without understanding what's going on, and there's gonna be some tension, for the person who's feeling up for it (no pun intended).

> **"Are we ever going to have sex again?**
>
> **What the heck happened to you?**
>
> **Am I not attractive to you anymore?**
>
> **Are you interested in somebody else?**
>
> **Hey, I have needs.**
>
> **We used to do this all the time."**

Whoo boy... are we having fun yet?

So there's no sex, there's no understanding of why, and now everyone's hurt, pissed, and feeling rejected. Oh good, let's pour some emotional "grease" on a physiological fire.

Low sex drive can be another freaking awful byproduct of this disease. And it's really common.

Let's take a flyby of the science.

The Science:

First off, you're not alone. **The American Medical Association (JAMA) study** reported on in February 1999, about 43% of women suffer sexual inadequacy [1] – that's pretty close to half!

Actually, they figured the number was probably higher.

Generally there are 4 areas of sexual issues: [2]

- **Lack of desire or interest in sex**

- **Inability to become aroused**

- **Inability to climax, or very slow to climax**

- **Pain during intercourse**

How many of the 43% have thyroid issues?

I don't know the exact number, but let's look at the connection between her thyroid malfunctioning, and her libido taking a nose dive.

Remember we learned ALL cells of our body have thyroid hormone receptors. Not enough thyroid hormone and the body's systems don't rev fast enough to do their job.

"Hypothyroidism is significantly linked to low libido. T3, the active form of thyroid hormone, is crucial for the proper functioning of cells and organs. Without T3, the reproductive system barely manages to inch forward.

Sex hormones suffer greatly, both at the ovarian level as well as in production at the hypothalamic and pituitary levels." [3] –
Author Stefani Ruper

"The adrenal glands that produce hormones that convert into the sex hormones are also slowed down… women can see decreased testosterone and estrogen levels." [4] –
Kent Holtorf, M.D.

That not just in her mind, it's in her body. It's the real deal.

1. Her thyroid levels being too low slows down the reproductive system

2. Then, it's common for women with thyroid issues to have other endocrine and hormone imbalances (estrogen, progesterone, and testosterone) [2]

So here's the equation. Low thyroid + maxed out adrenal glands = hormone imbalance. When this happens, the body conserves its energy for things like staying alive, and healing.

Sex isn't a priority for a body that's trying to heal, and that's likely why her sexual desire is not there.

Now that's just the physiological / body side of things. There can also be the psychological / mental game. Because, let's be honest guys, everyone comes to a relationship with some kind of baggage.

When you have statistics like, 1 in 5 women experience sexual abuse as a child,[5] this is already a sensitive area. Then you add on all the pressures of television, magazines, and social media, where almost every image is Photoshopped to perfection.

And then, on top of that, you add the concerns they have about their kids, and the finances, and the state of the world, and they're bringing all of that to the bedroom before they even were dealing with the thyroid issue. This isn't just a physical issue, this is a mental game, too.

Which brings me to...

My Story

So, how do you talk to a bunch of guys about your sex life?

Hmmm... well, Stacey and I have spent some 20 years coaching individuals or couples through some of their toughest relationship issues.

And guess what? No matter what the topic they came in the door with, what we ended up addressing was how that one thing ended up affecting their sex life and/or intimacy.

We need to talk about it honestly, because it's the real deal of what's going on in relationships. There's a lot of pain and misunderstanding out there, so it makes it an easy thing for me to open up about, especially if it helps a couple have hope, which can help stabilize a marriage, which can help make life better in a family, and the waves of impact go out from there.

So here we go...

In the beginning part of my dating and marriage to Stacey, sex was just wonderful.

We enjoyed each other, anytime we wanted, anywhere we could... yada yada, no need to go into specific details. It was fun, we were young and life was easy, uncomplicated, and full of opportunities.

Seven years into our marriage is when Stacey first started noticing odd symptoms, but didn't know what it was about – weight gain, feeling cold, brittle hair and skin issues.

We started seeing doctors who were doing their best to address the individual symptoms (at the time they didn't know it was Hashimoto's either). So, she wasn't feeling well, she was concerned, and she was gaining weight at rapid pace.

As the symptoms got worse and worse, and she had gained 100 pounds – reaching her heaviest weight of 270 pounds – her body wasn't the only thing changing; our sex life was changing too.

Now, you have to know, we didn't have a diagnosis, so all of this gaining weight and losing sex drive was falling into the mysterious realm of "I don't know what the hell is going on."

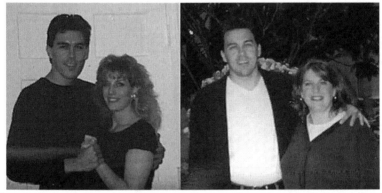

(The before and after photos. Wow, what the heck happened?)

She felt ugly and embarrassed. She was being treated differently by friends and family. So, she was already coming to the bedroom with feeling physically awful, and on top of it, was dealing with all these emotional hang-ups.

So guys, you need to know that sex is very much <u>a mind game</u> for women. While guys are easily ready for sex, women take longer to get in the mood.

"A woman's brain is the most crucial organ when it comes to sex - and a carefully chosen remark or gesture from a lover will prove far more effective." [6] – James Tozer

And so, for my woman who was sick with Hashimoto's...

- She was distracted

- She didn't feel well

- She was stressed out

- She felt unattractive

- She felt like she had lost her "old self"

- And... drum roll please, her hormones were all out of whack

When you do the math on how that might affect her mind and body, it's pretty simple to figure out why she wasn't in the mood.

I, on the other hand, didn't really change that much during this time. I was pretty much always ready for sex.

Go figure. Most guys are.

Having a wife who was significantly overweight <u>did</u> have an effect on our sex life. I would be lying if I said it didn't change anything. But sex still felt wonderful, and this was still the person I loved.

While we definitely started off our relationship with a lot of physical attraction, we also had spent almost a decade together, and had lived a fair amount of life up to that point. Our relationship, and my love for her was so much more than just how she looked.

If the shoe were on the other foot, and I had gained weight and now weighed **300** pounds – that would have an effect on her. And while that matters, it's not the biggest point when you're dealing with a serious health issue.

The bigger point was that she was not doing well physically. And if I wouldn't ask her for sex when she had the flu (or take it personally if she didn't want to) because she was trying to heal, so why couldn't I apply the same sensitivity here?

So, guys, that's our part of the game.

I'm going to share what my wife chose to do, and how she processed the consideration for her health and for our relationship.

She chose to have sex anyway.

Even though she didn't feel like it much of the time, it was her personal choice to connect with me that way. Here's the relevant quote from her book, **"You're Not Crazy and You're Not Alone"** in the chapter **Advice to My Younger "Me"**:

(Remember, this is Stacey talking to herself)

> "Okay, so here's the deal: you know how much you love sex? You may go through a time where you want to put a lock over your coochie and throw away the key. Stress, kids, and lack of sleep, as well as an underactive thyroid, may threaten to take the va-va-voom out of your bedroom.

It's okay. I'm telling you now: have sex anyway.

You'll still have a connecting, good time if you let yourself. It's good for your marriage. It's good for your soul. It's the closest thing to exercise you're going to be doing for a while and your guy loves it.

He's not looking at your cellulite. Hell, he can't even find the ketchup when it's the only thing in the fridge. No, really. Seriously, I read an article about how men don't even really see cellulite the way we do. I wish I had known that when I was your age.

So, you've gained some weight. So, you're not feeling 'into' it.

So, you're tired.

You're going to feel that way anyway until you sort out some of the health stuff, you might as well have some skin-on-skin time. It's good for your heart, it's going to give you some endorphins (which you probably desperately need), and heck, you may even lose some weight and get a nap out of the whole deal afterward.

This whole 'have sex anyway' can really be a good thing if you let it."

Now, I can imagine some guys standing up clapping, going...

"YEAH! Damn straight! She needs to help me. I have needs!"

All I can say is, *be careful here.*

My relationship is not yours. Our relational issues are likely different depending on how we were raised, our values, and what we both think is acceptable.

Do not print this up, shove it in her face, and say **"Rock and Stacey Robbins says we should have sex anyway"**.

Oh please don't.

Some women could be horrified to imagine having sex when they don't feel well, or have little desire.

Bottom line, you're going to have to work it out **together**. Talk to each other about it.

It is a relationship, after all.

Since sex for a woman is mostly in her mind, what would help her here?

(Yes, actually pause for a moment here and think what would help.)

I have some ideas.

Disclaimer
Of course, I have to start with the **aggravating disclaimer**. Captain Obvious says – everyone is different. What may work for one person, may not work for another; this goes for the mental game, and the treatment side of things.

It will take a commitment to work through your intimacy issues together. But if you are both working through it as partners, and give time and space for things to be "in process" – you will get to a better place sooo much faster than if you were fighting over this issue.

Ok, so you're in charge of your life, your relationship, and your results. Disclaimer over.

The Suggestions

The good news is that <u>you don't have to be perfect here</u>; trust me, just the sheer fact that you're reading this book gives you bonus points.

1. **Be present** – live in the reality of what your sex life is now. I understand that you wish it was the way it was back in the day, but don't live there – that's a sure way to keep frustrated.

2. **Be patient** – how I wish Hashimoto's were a quick and easy thing to fix. For libido it's a process – proper thyroid levels, adrenal repair, supplementation, and a less stressful life. Those are all the part of the road back to her health and a restored sex drive. That will likely take time to dial in. So, plan for the long distance road, and yet be open to it changing sooner.

3. **Be accepting** – let her know you love her and accept her body now. Even if she doesn't look the way she used to, or the way you wished she did, trust me – you're not the only one dealing with dashed dreams and harsh realities right now; she's likely going through it too. You're both having to adjust, why not do it together? Let go of being things being perfect. Life just is what it is right now. Perfection = stress, and she doesn't need more stress right now.

4. **Find other ways to be intimate** – I really hope this is not a brand new thought for you.

   Remember how most of sex for women is in their mind? Think about when you were first seeing, or dating your woman. You probably talked a lot together, maybe went out to dinner. Maybe you played card games, or went on walks in the park. Laughing together, holding hands, talking for hours – many of these were probably part of your early relationship.

   Of course, there was sex too (**yessir!**), but that wasn't all of your relationship, was it? There's something to just even holding each other on a comfy couch and watching a fun video.

   Sometimes she only has enough energy to cover the basics, and doing something as mundane as grocery shopping together can be a fun time to talk and be together.

   Have her listen to what her body can handle, and find other creative ways to build intimacy.

5. **Make the bedroom a peaceful place instead of a "pressure to have sex or an orgasm place"** – remember the whole juicy hamburger when you have the flu example?

   How would you like food to be shoved in your face when you're sick?

   How would you like to be pressured to eat it?

   You'd want to get away from that person.

   Don't be that person.

6. **Invest in her** – this is the *new* foreplay. It's the proof that you love her for better or worse, and is the warm up for more intimacy.

   What I hear from other Hashimoto's women on my wife's Facebook site is that it can be small acts of kindness that make a big difference.

   I know we can get stuck for ideas, so here are a few...

   - Ask how she's doing (and really listen to the answer)
   - Give her a back rub
   - Take her to the doctor's appointment (and actually pay attention)
   - Read up on anything Hashimoto's or health related
   - Make sure she's taking her meds, or supplements
   - Hire someone to do the cleaning
   - Watch a video of her/your favorite comedian
   - Go down the greeting card aisle, and read the funny cards to each other
   - Have a weekly time of reviewing her health plan
   - Wild Idea – ask her!

   I want you to win, so here's one of my best lines, that I say sincerely, that really hits it out of the park:

   "Honey... (dramatic pause)

   Is there anything I can do for you right now?"

7. **Get counseling / coaching** – this of course, is optional. But if you're still having problems that you can't break through together, sometimes a counselor or coach can help you see what you can't see.

   Imagine you're both in a maze and can't find the exit. You're feel stuck, and you don't know where to go.

   Now imagine someone above the maze, who can see you where you are and how to direct you to where you want to be. That's what coaching provides: perspective, guidance and support. Find someone competent and let them help you.

   If you're interested in coaching from Stacey and/or me, go to **www.marriedtohashimotos.com/coaching** for more details. We do individual and couples coaching and would be honored to help you navigate this maze.

   You know what all this does? It gives her *hope*. Because when you invest in her, you're telling her that you believe she can get better, and that you'll have a future together. That is something she's probably not getting anywhere else.

   That is pure gold, and is perfect foreplay.

   Be encouraged, there is hope. Things can get better.

   It will take investment, but it's more than worth it.

   For me and my wife, we found that once her health was more in order, our sex picked up again.

So guys, this is not rocket science...

1. You want to have sex, and she wants to get better

2. Help her get better, and you'll likely get more sex

(Can't click on these? Well, this is just a book. Search online for the title, or go to **www.marriedtohashimotos.com/booklinks** for all of the links listed here, plus more.)

Referenced articles:

1. **Sexual Dysfunction in the United States: Prevalence and Predictors**
   http://www.ncbi.nlm.nih.gov/pubmed/10022110

2. **Sexual Dysfunction and Thyroid Disease Solutions**
   https://www.verywell.com/low-sex-drive-and-thyroid-disease-hypothyroidism-3231814

3. **Paleo And Sex: How To Have A Ravenous And Kickass Female Libido**
   http://paleoforwomen.com/paleo-and-sex-how-to-have-a-ravenous-and-kickass-female-libido

4. **Thyroid Disease And Low Libido**
   https://www.holtorfmed.com/thyroid-disease-and-low-libido

5. **Child Sexual Abuse Statistics**
   https://victimsofcrime.org/media/reporting-on-child-sexual-abuse/child-sexual-abuse-statistics

6. **Sex All in the Mind for Women**
   http://www.dailymail.co.uk/femail/article-299254/Sex-mind-women.html

Related articles:

- **9 Ways to Revive Your Libido with Hypothyroidism + 7 Libido Boosting Foods**
  https://drbrighten.com/9-ways-to-revive-your-libido-with-hypothyroidism-7-libido-boosting-foods

- **Can Natural Thyroid Treatments Improve Your Sex Life?**
  http://www.naturalendocrinesolutions.com/articles/can-natural-thyroid-treatments-improve-your-sex-life

- **Thyroid May Cause Sexual Problems**
  http://www.webmd.com/women/news/20020321/thyroid-may-cause-sexual-problems

- **Intimacy Without Intercourse**
  http://www.healthywomen.org/content/article/intimacy-without-intercourse?context=ages-and-stages/10191

- **9 Simple Ways To Build Intimacy and Protect Any Long-Term Relationship**
  http://www.bustle.com/articles/44368-9-simple-ways-to-build-intimacy-and-protect-any-long-term-relationship

Closing Fireside
Chat with Rock

Wow. Congratulations. You did it.

Again, BIG HIGH FIVE for even picking up this book, because many don't and just kind of wing it or bury their head in the sand.

I know we covered a lot of ground, but the crazy thing is – this was the shorter version. I tried to keep it as streamlined as possible for you.

I imagined that you were as overwhelmed as I was when this whole thing entered my world so... there you go.

Hey, do me a favor. I want to hear from you and get your feedback. What hit you and what you want to hear more of? This is not the end of the conversation.

You can reach me: **contact@marriedtohashimotos.com.** And while you're at it, go to **ww.marriedtohashimotos.com** and sign up for updates. I'll keep that guy wisdom coming direct to your inbox.

Throw me your questions and I'll turn them into blog Question and Answer aticles.

And if you need even more help, **set up a one-on-one coaching session** with me, or even a **couples session** for you and your woman and my wife and I. We're here to help you win at this health partnership journey.

I know you can do this. Now you have some good tools to help you build the health and life you want for you, your woman, and your family (if you have one).

Just remember: You're not alone.

You've got this.

We're in this together.

Ciao,

You Rock!

(Gratitudes)

I couldn't have done this without the help of friends who believed in me, even though I know I make them a little crazy. I know... it's a gift.

David Trotter – "mind blown" by your generosity and the big life game you play. You da man. Thank you.

Michael and Izabella Wentz – you guys have been such an inspiring example of a power couple making a positive difference in the world. Thank you so much for your friendship and for being just really cool people.

Dana Trentini – well, well Dana. This whole book adventure really took off thanks to you sharing my post. I love that we're connected and get to help women, men, and their families. Thank you!

Irene Dunlap – Rene! OMG. This is just the thank you for the editing help, but you've been such a huge part of our family's life for 20 years. Mille grazie!

Angela Ippolito and **Dave Cottam** – Wowza guys, your advocacy and help getting us across the U.S. and to the Italian promised land set the stage for this book being possible. Love you guys, and I'm so looking forward to some family fun with you all soon.

Special shout out to the **Girlfriends' Guide to Hashimoto's Facebook Group** that my wife Stacey started. You gals were so supportive – giving input, cheering me on, and telling your other girlfriends about this book.

And of course to my family...

Caleb Robbins – Mr. Big Man. Almost as tall as me (but not there yet!) I'm so proud of you, and am so thankful that you helped me cross the finish line with this by just being an awesome, and easy help to our family. Love you KK.

Seth Robbins – Captain Awesome Junior. You just keep getting more and more wise and handsome. I appreciate how you helped keep our home clean, and worked with your bro to take care of things when I was locked in the "man cave" writing. So proud of who you truly are in the world. Big love to you Sefferson.

And finally to my...

Stacey

... my amazing wife, life partner, mother of my kiddos, personal chef, Italian lover, Yahtzee partner, and one wonderfully wise, funny, and "refreshing" dance partner in life.

I could just keep on writing, and writing. Too much to cover here other than... thank you for believing in me, and supporting me.

I love you so.

Made in the USA
Middletown, DE
21 October 2020